T0247911

Defying Death

Medicine's Journey Toward Immortality

Bruno Leone and Michael A. Leone

For more information, contact:
ReferencePoint Press, Inc.
PO Box 27779
San Diego, CA 92198
www.ReferencePointPress.com

cover: Red Line Editorial
12: Look and Learn/Bridgeman Images
27: NPL-DeA Picture Library/Bridgeman Library
45: Red Line Editorial
78: Aflo Co. LTD./Alamy Stock Photo
94: dpa picture alliance/Alamy Stock Photo
125: MattLphotography/Shutterstock.com

LIBRARY OF CONGRESS CATALOGING-IN-PUBLICATION DATA

Names: Leone, Bruno, 1939-author. | Leone, Michael A., author.

Title: Defying death: medicine's journey toward immortality / by Bruno J. Leone and
    Michael A. Leone.

Description: San Diego, CA: ReferencePoint Press, Inc., 2024. | Includes bibliographical
    references and index.

Identifiers: LCCN 2022054715 (print) | LCCN 2022054716 (eBook) | ISBN
    9781678205140 (hardcover) | ISBN 9781678205157 (eBook)

Subjects: LCSH: Longevity--Juvenile literature. | Medicine, Preventive--History--
    Juvenile literature. | Aging--Prevention--Juvenile literature. | Life expectancy--Juvenile
    literature.

Classification: LCC RA776.75.L456 2024 (print) | LCC RA776.75 (eBook) | DDC 613.2-
    -dc23/eng/20221223

LC record available at https://lccn.loc.gov/2022054715

LC eBook record available at https://lccn.loc.gov/2022054716

Contents

Prologue

Increases in human life expectancy have over the centuries relied in large part on the effectiveness of medical science's attempts to prevent the occurrence of disease or to successfully treat disease when it does occur. For millennia, healers of all types have labored tirelessly in their efforts to prolong life. Indeed, one of the universal responsibilities all doctors tacitly acknowledge is to keep their patients alive and well for as long as is humanly possible. This axiom has weathered the storms and vicissitudes of history in all parts of the globe. It has been embraced by Chinese acupuncturists, Siberian shamans, Navajo medicine men, medieval bloodletters, and the Memorial Sloan Kettering Cancer Center—as well as the "Father of Medicine," the classical Greek Hippocrates (ca. 460 BCE–ca. 375 BCE), who admonished his students to "help the sick" and to "do no harm." The fact that all practitioners of the healing arts, although representative of different cultures and periods in history, are similarly committed to maintaining the well-being of their patients speaks to a belief that humanity can overcome some factors that otherwise would shorten life spans. All healers, then, answer in their own way to the same call to prolong human life.

Despite working within the limits of what current medical practices can achieve, extending a patient's life has taken on a far greater potential in the world of twenty-first-century medicine. As ever-improving drugs, therapeutic and surgical procedures, and diagnostic tools become available to the public, patient longevity typically follows suit. Demographic studies of life expectancy generally depict upward trends at times when science, especially medical science, is on the ascendancy. And during those valued moments when a particular medical discovery surfaces that proves to be applicable and effective far beyond its original expectations, a comparable increase in life expectancy will be the telltale outcome.

Such a response followed the fortuitous discovery of penicillin in 1929. An antibiotic used in the treatment of bacterial infections, penicillin enjoyed and continues to enjoy extensive and unparalleled success when properly prescribed. "Prior to this discovery," Massachusetts General Hospital's Nicole McFarlane points out, "infections such as bacterial endocarditis, bacterial meningitis, and pneumococcal pneumonia were often deadly. Penicillin's discovery then sparked a new era of medicine where doctors finally held a powerful tool in their hands to stop the spread and fatality of infectious diseases."[1]

In addition to antibiotics, vaccines, and other key medical discoveries that increased human life spans, a second public health trend contributed significantly to that prolonged longevity—namely, the rise in sanitary practices beginning in the late 1800s and early 1900s. This included the habitual employment of simple measures such as handwashing, use of antiseptics in operations and other medical procedures, and other forms of cleanliness. Indeed, public sanitary advances are often driven by and/or beholden to medical research and invention, and the two have repeatedly seemed to springboard off one another over the past couple of centuries, steadily increasing human longevity in the process.

Moreover, medical advances that were once the subject of science fiction are now the building blocks of tomorrow's breakthroughs. Physicians treat not only the body—the *corpus*—of their patients but also the cells and subcellular organelles residing within. Also, we live in an age of modern medicine that operates on the molecular level. If cellular degeneration, an important cause of aging, ever becomes just another disease to be treated, perhaps we can anticipate life expectancy to experience double- and triple-digit increases, which conceivably would carry humanity's life span even beyond that which nature has thus far allotted. And to highlight the obvious, we have only taken our first steps on the path to a brave new era in modern medicine.

Defying Death: Medicine's Journey Toward Immortality is an attempt to outline where medicine has traveled in the past and to chart where it may be heading in the future. More specifically, this work endeavors to illustrate how advances in modern medical technology often leave in their wake increases in human life expectancy. In the words of researchers at the United Kingdom's Tony Blair Institute of Global Change, "One of humanity's greatest success stories of the past century is the increase in global life expectancy as a result of the social and medical advancements that have dramatically improved basic living conditions and reduced vulnerability to infectious diseases."[2]

As we ponder this exciting odyssey in medical science, one telling question begs to be answered: is this a story without an ending? That is, will every new century or millennium fashion its own singular contribution to the number of years each human's body and mind can expect to survive? And will this continue indefinitely? Or does the story of humanity reach a chapter (or perhaps a "grand finale") in which the body will no longer be needed? Could it be that the collective consciousness of humanity will reside and hopefully even flourish on the hard drive of a computer (or some other such device), creating an almost endless future—one that a small but steadily growing number of distinguished scientists, scholars, and transhumanists believe is humanity's ultimate fate?

Notes

1. Nicole McFarlane, "The History of Penicillin," Allergy and Asthma Center of Boston, February 4, 2020. www.allergyasthmaboston.com.
2. Karen Hooper et al., "Live Longer or Healthier? The Science That Is Making Both Possible," Tony Blair Institute for Global Change, November 5, 2021. https://institute.global.

Part I

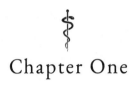

Chapter One

The Medicine of Yesterday

The road that has taken us to our current life expectancy has been painfully long, and we, the travelers, have been weighed down by disease and ignorance. Throughout the greater part of human history, doctors and other practitioners of the healing arts have been largely unsuccessful at realizing all—or at times even part—of their quest to extend the lives of their patients. As a result, incalculable numbers of human beings, generation upon generation, have faced predictably early deaths. Although demographic estimates tend to vary and often lack accuracy because of their imprecise and contingent nature, most scientists and medical historians would likely agree that the archaeological and historical records of humanity for virtually all but the past three or four centuries reveal a life expectancy falling somewhere between thirty and forty-five years. However, this does not mean that human beings of the past never lived longer than that. Verifiable scientific and historical evidence indicates that many did enjoy reasonably long lives. As Australian archaeologist Christine Cave points out, "The

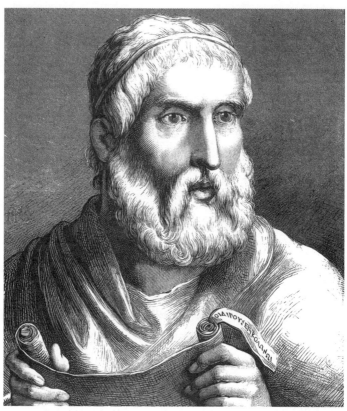

Ancient Greek playwright Sophocles is believed to have lived to the age of ninety.

ancient Greeks classed old age among the divine curses, and their tombstones attest to survival [of some individuals] well past 80 years."[1] In fact, among the classical Greeks, some of whose ages have been reliably estimated by historians, the great scholar and thinker Plato lived to be about eighty; the noted playwright Euripides died at age eighty-one; and Euripides's fellow tragedian Sophocles made it to the proverbial ripe old age of ninety. Nevertheless, on average a statistically significant percentage of people born each year in ancient times would not live long enough to celebrate their thirtieth birthdays.

One of the foremost reasons for such unfavorable data is that until the dawn of the modern era of medicine, all knowledge and understanding of the internal parts of the human body and the mechanisms guiding it were misunderstood or at best very limited. Although doctors of all types attempted to define and describe the human body and its respective systems, their efforts yielded no meaningful explanations of what kept the human body alive, well, and functioning. Under those circumstances, the diagnosis and treatment of patients' illnesses essentially were akin to a "shot in the dark." Moreover, questions related to the cellular composition and purpose of major organs like the brain, heart, lungs, liver, and kidneys or body fluids like lymph and blood were generally not addressed or were commonly misinterpreted.

To illustrate, Isidore of Seville (560–636 CE), a renowned Spanish medieval scholar and bishop, composed a multivolume encyclopedia that attempted to reveal and explain much of the existing scientific and nonscientific knowledge of his day. Entitled *Etymologiae* (meaning "the study of word origins"), the medical portion of his work was filled with illogical assumptions, inaccuracies, and ludicrous or superstitious statements. His almost whimsical explanation for the situation of the human anus, for instance, was that "the posterior parts [of the body] are indeed so named because they are behind, turned away from the face, lest we be offended by the sight as we empty our bowels."[2] Regarding the role of blood in the human body, Isidore claimed that the young possess an inexhaustible supply. But as we age, he notes, "physicians say that the blood supply is diminished" and that the decreased amount of blood causes "tremor[s] to occur in the elderly." Following this string of inexactitudes, Isidore concluded by stating that "properly, blood is controlled by the soul."[3] It is noteworthy that his *Etymologiae* was one of the most frequently consulted reference works in the Middle Ages. And even more significant, it was not at all atypical. Indeed, it was quite illustrative of many of the encyclopedic works circulating among and referenced by scholars throughout the ancient and medieval worlds.

A Cosmos of Microscopic Creatures

By far, however, the most consequential shortcoming of premodern medicine was the fact that doctors (along with the rest of humanity) were totally unaware of the existence of microbes that both surround and reside within the human body. Invisible to the naked eye, this cosmos of living creatures inhabits the earth in seemingly endless numbers. Referred to collectively as "germs," among others, the organisms include bacteria, viruses, and protozoa and have been responsible for more premature deaths than any other single factor, including warfare. And because germs were unseen and therefore unsuspected, physicians understandably had no reason to attempt to treat them or to seek to avoid them.

As a result, what is commonly referred to today as "germ theory" was nowhere to be found in any medical literature written prior to the past three hundred years. In her 2007 book, *Deadly Companions: How Microbes Shaped Our History*, Dorothy H. Crawford, professor of medical microbiology at the University of Edinburgh, stresses the appalling and inevitable consequences resulting from this ignorance of germ theory. She writes:

> Although through the ages, many theories emerged to explain phenomena [such as epidemics and individual infectious diseases; the theories] were generally misguided, and the treatments they invoked usually did more harm than good. . . . In fact, right up until the eighteenth century most herbal remedies used by doctors . . . contained no active ingredients . . . [and] the best advice a doctor could offer during epidemics was to flee or pray (or both).[4]

Until medicine recognized the existence of germs and their ability to cause varying degrees of harm to the human body—especially death—the situation described by Crawford accounted significantly for the brevity of the human life span.

New Methods of Reasoning and Experimentation

But that recognition would eventually come and with it a promise destined to transform human history. The beginning of the modern age in European history gave birth to an intellectual phenomenon that would radically alter the nature and outcomes of virtually all the sciences, especially medicine. During the sixteenth and seventeenth centuries, numerous obsolete and flawed ideas that had dominated pedagogy gradually began to yield to dramatically unique patterns of learning. Following on the gains of the European Renaissance (ca. 1350–ca. 1600), Western thinkers turned to methods of reasoning and experimentation first recorded by the ancient Greeks and carried through Roman and eventually medieval times. Some even borrowed from Arabic thought via the remnants of the Byzantine Empire. These practices had long remained effectively dormant because the early medieval world lacked the capability to reproduce and disseminate them. Kept alive in scattered monasteries and other such remote repositories, these ancient processes of scientific inquiry only came to light with the invention of printing with movable type in the mid-1400s. Empiricism (the idea that all knowledge derives from detection by the senses), championed by English philosopher and statesman Francis Bacon (1561–1626), gave shape to a scientific method based on observation, inductive reasoning, and repeated experimentation. Perception, Bacon asserted, "all depends on keeping the eye steadily fixed upon the facts of nature and so receiving their images simply as they are."[5] This transformation proved a turning point in history, one of those rare and defining periods in time when great minds set sail upon uncharted waters and providentially land on rich, fruitful shores. Historians appropriately have labeled this epoch of profound change the Scientific Revolution.

The great transformation of human thought loosened the intellectual and cultural shackles of European life. Philosophers, mathematicians, scientists, and even artists began applying novel methods of study to expose and explore the mysteries of the physical and biological worlds through direct observation. Reasoned and critical thinking about the natural world, along with objective experimentation, replaced the blind acceptance of hidebound ancient authorities. According to a leading historian of the Scientific Revolution, Kathryn Wolford:

> A monumental shift in what constituted
> evidence for truth was under way. Not only

did renaissance artisans create lenses to see, tools to measure, and artworks to replicate the natural world, but by the sixteenth century, they began to publish philosophical treatises asserting that through the imitation and reproduction of nature in their arts, they were able to achieve a state of direct engagement with nature. Rather than taking knowledge from ancient sources, they argued that true knowledge came from direct experience.[6]

As a result, prejudicial ideas that typified the Dark Ages (as the Middle Ages was sometimes referenced) gave way to innovative and unbiased concepts. Indeed, larger numbers of philosophers and scientists finally felt compelled to question and often completely revise centuries-old axioms and assumptions about nature and the universe, including numerous medical concepts. Not only were many such assumptions in error, but leading thinkers began to assert that these faulty beliefs were also serious obstacles to genuine progress and discovery.

Meanwhile, Far to the East

What the vast majority of Europeans in the period spanning ca. 1350 to 1600, including most of the emerging scientists, did not know was that they were not the only humans destined to make crucial new medical discoveries. Indeed, by that time, thousands of miles to the east, Chinese healers had developed medical knowledge in a number of ways similar in scope to that of Europe. Although the Chinese did not create an overall scientific revolution, they had a long tradition of logical and effective medical advancements.

Much of that Chinese medical lore was based on a pivotal document that appeared sometime between 300 and 100 BCE—the *Huangdi Neijing*, roughly translated as *The Inner Canon of the Yellow Emperor*. Before its appearance, the Chinese had assumed that disease was caused either by demons or by angry ancestors placing curses on their descendants. In contrast, the *Huangdi Neijing*, whose authorship remains unknown, held that there are physical causes for illness, especially various bodily imbalances. In this way early Chinese medical thought paralleled that of a number of ancient Greek physicians. The *Huangdi Neijing*, which became the leading basis for later Chinese medicine, described various aspects of human anatomy, the circulation of the blood, and a number of apparently effective treatments for sick people, prominent among them acupuncture.

Later Chinese doctors expanded such ideas, adding new medical knowledge. Hua Tuo (ca. 110–208 CE), for example, invented an anesthetic made from cannabis that caused a patient to briefly lose consciousness, making painless operations possible. Later still, Sun Simiao (ca. 581–682 CE) wrote several medical treatises, notably about growing medical herbs and treating illnesses associated with women. In Sun's own words, "The reason there are separate prescriptions for women is that they get pregnant, give birth, and suffer from uterine damage. This is why women's disorders are ten times more difficult to cure than those of males."[7]

A Refreshing Intellectual Climate

Historians of science point out that many of the conclusions reached by medieval Chinese and European physicians about diagnosing and treating certain illnesses were surprisingly similar. Yet the two medical systems seem to have developed independently of each other. Importantly, the most basic of those resemblances was that both traditions primarily sought to keep patients healthy, which at times had the fortunate by-product of allowing them to live longer. To humankind's good fortune, such advances in medicine relieved human suffering to one degree or another in two large geographical spheres separated by many vast plains and mountain ranges. Perhaps in part by chance, it was in the westernmost of those two regions—Europe—that the vanguard of new medical discoveries and changes spawned by the Scientific Revolution took root and flourished in this refreshing intellectual climate. Andreas Vesalius (1514–1564) was one of the pioneers of that series of advances. A Flemish (modern-day Belgian) physician, he brought clarity and new life to his profession with the publication of an anatomy textbook unlike any previously written. Entitled *De Humani Corporis Fabrica* (*On the Fabric of the Human Body*, 1543), the seven-volume work derived from observations of human dissections that he performed while lecturing at the University of Padua in Italy. Unknown to their readers, earlier anatomy books, such as the widely read text written by the Greco-Roman physician Galen (129 CE–ca. 216), based their portrayals of the human body on the dissection of animals, most frequently pigs, dogs, sheep, and apes. Some scholars believe this was the result of a cultural or legal prohibition against human dissection in ancient Rome; others point out that it might also be attributable to an inadequate supply of corpses to study in that era. Regardless, Galen's work had its limits. For instance, because he could not dissect humans, he based most of his theories of human anatomy on comparisons and analogies to the many animals he was able to dissect. And many of his assumptions made in such comparisons were incorrect.

Vesalius respected Galen's medical pursuits, but he believed surgeons and scientists had to work hands-on with the subject of their study. To accompany his revelations in *De Humani Corporis Fabrica*, Vesalius commissioned illustrations that were without equal and set a standard for anatomical drawings produced before the advent of photography. His work garnered him much fame and an appointment as a physician to Charles V (1500–1558), the Holy Roman emperor, in 1543.

In the tradition of Vesalius, English physician William Harvey (1578–1657) made a series of landmark discoveries regarding the nature and structure of the human circulatory system. Prior to Harvey most physicians accepted that blood was produced in the liver from food stored there by the body. It then passed from the liver into the heart, where it was heated. Once sufficiently heated, it was able to flow into veins, which in turn distributed the nutrient-rich blood throughout the body.

Contrary to this prevailing orthodoxy, Harvey was able to demonstrate that the heart, not the liver, was the central organ in the cardiovascular system. He further proved that it was not heat but rather the heart's pumping action that caused blood to be passed along through its various chambers and valves before being ejected into the general circulation, where it could then nourish the entire body. He determined that the arterial system (arteries) carried renewed blood throughout the body while the venous system (veins) returned blood to the heart, thereby completing the circulatory process. Harvey stated with no small measure of confidence:

I surveyed my mass of evidence, whether
derived from vivisections, and my various
reflections on them, or from the study of
the ventricles of the heart and the vessels
that enter into and issue from them . . .
or from observing the arrangement and
intricate structure of the valves in particular, and of the other parts of the heart in
general . . . [and] I began to think whether
there might not be A MOTION, AS IT
WERE, IN A CIRCLE. Now this I after-
wards found to be true; and I finally saw
that the blood, forced by the action of the
left ventricle into the arteries, was distributed to the body at large, and its several parts,
in the same manner as it is sent through
the lungs, impelled by the right ventricle
into the pulmonary artery, and that it then
passed through the veins and along the
vena cava, and so round to the left ventricle
in the manner already indicated. This motion we may be allowed to call circular.[8]

Through such meticulous and logical observation,
along with mathematical calculations, Harvey document-
ed these ideas and more in his 1628 book entitled *Exerci-
tatio Anatomica de Motu Cordis et Sanguinis in Animalibus*

(*Anatomical Study of the Motion of the Heart and of the Blood in Animals*). One of the landmark books in the history of the healing arts, it was initially rejected by conservative physicians, especially those who attributed a spiritual quality to the heart. Harvey viewed the heart as an organic pump that kept people alive, not the seat of the soul, as Aristotle had believed. Harvey insisted, "The heart of animals [and human beings] is the foundation of their life, the sovereign of everything within them, the sun of their microcosm, that upon which all growth depends, from which all power proceeds."[9] By the end of his life, though, his studies on the circulatory system were widely known and largely accepted, and his *De Motu Cordis* proved to be a cornerstone of modern medicine.

Vesalius and Harvey were but two of a growing number of physicians who played leading roles during the dawn of modern medicine, setting the scene for what would eventually be studies and theories about human longevity. Another was Philippus Aureolus Theophrastus Bombastus von Hohenheim, more commonly known as Paracelsus (1493–1541). A German Swiss doctor and philosopher, he highlighted the importance of chemistry in medicine. Ambroise Paré (1510–1590), a gifted French surgeon, developed numerous surgical techniques (such as clamping off surgically-severed blood vessels to prevent hemorrhaging), several of which are still being used today. Many consider him to be the father of modern surgery. Also, studies in microscopic anatomy by Marcello Malpighi (1628–1694), an Italian biologist, laid the foundation for the fields of embryology and physiology. Meanwhile, Thomas Sydenham (1624–1689) has been long recognized as the founder of clinical medicine and epidemiology and is often referred to as the "English Hippocrates." And Antonio Benivieni (1443–1502), a Florentine surgeon, dissected deceased patients to help determine the cause of their deaths. Some of his procedures are still employed today in autopsies, earning him the title of father of pathologic anatomy. In addition, there was Nils Rosén von Rosenstein (1706–1773), a Swedish physician who in 1752 wrote *The Diseases of Children and Their Remedies*, a systematic textbook covering the symptoms, pathology, and treatment of a broad spectrum of childhood diseases. His text was the first modern work of its kind and helped establish pediatrics as a medical specialty.

Humanity was the ultimate beneficiary of this list of groundbreaking physicians and scientists whose guiding principle, empiricism, dictated that reason, experience, observation, and experimentation be central to the study of the sciences in the West. The wide-ranging discoveries and advances achieved during the Scientific Revolution ensured that antiquated beliefs and procedures were doomed. The medical validity of practices such as bloodletting—using leeches to rebalance the four bodily humors—and corpse medicine—consuming the blood of someone who recently passed away to revitalize the spirit—was increasingly questioned.

Key Advances in Bacteriology

Ultimately, the key to longevity that this historical period bestowed upon humanity lies in the widespread adoption of empiricism, or the need for evidence to support and guide a practice. Moreover, the Scientific Revolution helped lay the foundation for the decades of discoveries that followed. These discoveries would culminate in the advances in bacteriology that largely defined nineteenth- and twentieth-century medicine and their contribution to human longevity. And, finally, the hour was approaching when the earth's most pervasive killers, infectious microbes, would pose a substantially smaller threat to humanity.

The existence of virulent germs had been suspected—although never proved—for some time. For example, Girolamo Fracastoro (ca. 1478–1553), a physician from Verona, Italy, published a book in 1546 entitled *On Contagion and Contagious Diseases*. Fracastoro, a true visionary, anticipated the germ theory of infectious diseases by three centuries. He attributed the cause of epidemics and diseases like bubonic plague, smallpox, and measles to something he identified as *seminaria*, or seeds. And although the first compound microscope was not invented until nearly fifty years after his death, he nonetheless correctly theorized that seminaria existed and spread among their human hosts in three ways. One way, he said, consisted of "infection by contact only." The second method he predicted by which germs spread was "infection by contact and by fomites." Fracastoro identified these fomites as "such things as clothes, linen, etc., which although not themselves corrupt, can nevertheless foster the *essential seeds* of the contagion and thus cause infection." Third, he went on, "there is another class of infection which acts not only by contact and by fomites but can also be transmitted from a distance (inhaled without direct contact). Such are the pestilential fevers (Bubonic Plague), phthisis (airborne diseases like Tuberculosis) . . . [and] variola (smallpox) and their like."[10]

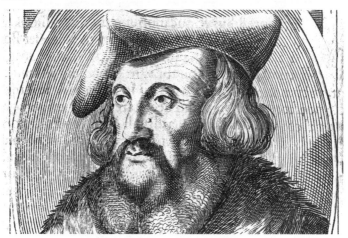

Portrait of Girolamo Fracastoro created in 1640.

Whereas Fracastoro's observations were theoretical in nature and at best revealed the shrewd and inductive mind associated with the Scientific Revolution, it was not until the seventeenth century that a major leap was taken that would eventually lead to the empirical recognition of the germ theory of disease. Antonie van Leeuwenhoek (1632–1723), an inspector of weights and measures for the town of Delft in the Netherlands, took up as a hobby the grinding of glass lenses to be used in microscopes. Although microscopes had been in use for nearly a half century before Van Leeuwenhoek was born, their lens quality was poor and, accordingly, their magnification was very limited. His lenses, on the other hand, magnified objects twenty to thirty times greater than earlier ones and thus were able to dramatically reduce the chasm separating the visible from the invisible world. He observed what some scientists, including Fracastoro, had only inferred—verification of the existence of seemingly countless living microscopic organisms.

Van Leeuwenhoek and His Microscope

Van Leeuwenhoek named his microbial discovery *animalcules*, or "tiny animals." In time it became apparent to him that his animalcules were omnipresent. They resided in the air he breathed, on the ground on which he walked, in the water he drank, on his neighbor's teeth, and much to his astonishment, in his own feces. They were also, by his estimation, incredibly numerous. In 1683 he wrote of his suspicion that "all the people living in our United Netherlands are not as many as the living animals that I carry in my own mouth this very day."[11] Van Leeuwenhoek further noticed that the little creatures differed in size and shape. "Their bodies," he said, were "somewhat longer than broad, and their belly, which [is] flat-like, furnished with sundry little paws wherewith they make such a stir in the clear medium . . . that you might even fancy you saw a pissabed [wood louse] running up against a wall."[12]

Such distinctiveness in shape of the animalcules motivated Van Leeuwenhoek to have them sketched by an artist. Over time, he published nearly four hundred illustrations of his "tiny animals." As word of Van Leeuwenhoek's discovery spread, so also did the accolades he regularly received from many of Europe's foremost scientists. In recognition of his achievement, he was elected to membership in two of the Western world's most prestigious scientific organizations—England's Royal Society and the French Academy of Sciences (both of which remain active today).

Ironically, the issue of causality completely eluded Van Leeuwenhoek. He never considered the likelihood of a cause-and-effect relationship between the invisible world of his "tiny animals" and the visible world of epidemics and individual diseases; and not surprisingly, there is no

indication that any of the learned scientists who mar-
veled at his discovery ever explored the possibility of a
causal connection. The fact is that no one at the time had
any reason to presume an association existed between microbes and disease. For one thing, Van Leeuwenhoek, his
friends and neighbors, and countless other people whom
he encountered regularly showed no signs of illness despite being exposed daily to the animalcules.

But there was a more compelling reason for regarding
the microscopic organisms as little more than benign
residents of the global community. For over fifteen
hundred years, many physicians and educated laymen
generally attributed the source of all contagious diseases
to a phenomenon called miasma (from the Greek word
for "pollution"), a mist or vapor that supposedly trans-
ported noxious impurities through the air. Miasmatic
fogs were said to draw their lethal essence from putre-
fying organic matter (such as rotting vegetation and
decomposing animal and human flesh) as they stealthily
passed through fields, villages, and towns. It was believed
that a person became infected if the miasma's deadly
cargo gained entrance into his or her body and disrupted
its vital functions. And although the miasma theory of
contagion, without proof or merit, remained prominent
for well over fifteen hundred years, it quickly faded into
history under the mountain of evidence supporting
germ theory, which, fortunately for humanity, came to

dominate medical science in the nineteenth and twentieth centuries. In the process, that veritable explosion of knowledge about germs and their connection to disease would also constitute an important next step toward the provocative and compelling goal of achieving human life extension.

Notes

1. Christine Cave, "Think Everyone Died Young in Ancient Societies? Think Again," Aeon, July 9, 2018. https://aeon.co.

2. Quoted in Plinio Prioreschi, *A History of Medicine*. Omaha, NE: Horatius, 2003, p. 151.

3. Quoted in Edward Grant, ed., *A Sourcebook in Medical Science*. Cambridge, MA: Harvard University Press, 1974, p. 723.

4. Dorothy H. Crawford, *Deadly Companions: How Microbes Shaped Our History*. New York: Oxford University, 2009, p. 183.

5. Quoted in Philip C.E. Stamp, University of British Columbia, "The 'Experimental Philosophy': Francis Bacon (1561–1626 AD)." https://phas.ubc.ca.

6. Kathryn Wolford, "A-Level: Francis Bacon and the Scientific Revolution," Smarthistory, July 20, 2017. https://smarthistory.org.

7. Quoted in Stephen Mortlock, "A History of Chinese Medicine," Biomedical Scientist, September 3, 2020. https://thebiomedicalscientist.net.

8. Quoted in Internet History Sourcebooks Project, "On the Motion of the Heart, Excerpts," 2021. https://sourcebooks.fordham.edu.

9. Quoted in Internet History Sourcebooks Project, "On the Motion of the Heart, Excerpts."

10. Girolamo Fracastoro, "On Contagion, Contagious Diseases and Their Cure," in *Source Book of Medical History*, ed. Logan Clendening. New York: Dover, 1942, pp. 107–109.

11. Quoted in Charles-Edward Winslow, *The Conquest of Epidemic Disease*. Madison: University of Wisconsin Press, 1980, p. 158.

12. Quoted in Alan L. Gillen and Douglas Oliver, "Antony van Leeuwenhoek: Creation 'Magnified' Through His Magnificent Microscopes," Answers in Genesis, August 15, 2012. https://answersingenesis.org.

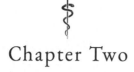

Chapter Two

The Medicine of Today

The nineteenth and twentieth centuries ushered in many of the most celebrated advances in medical therapeutics. And it was germ theory, more than any other discovery thus far, that succeeded in bridging the chasm of ignorance that separated modern medicine from its medieval and ancient predecessors. It also did more to prolong human life than any other medical discovery up to that time or since. In part this was because over time, knowledge of germs' destructive properties allowed doctors to treat or cure many diseases, and some of those who were saved went on to live far longer than they would have otherwise. Moreover, in the late nineteenth and early twentieth centuries, an ever-growing number of prominent doctors and scientists throughout the world gained attention and notoriety, not only in scientific journals but also in the popular press for their contributions to and acceptance of germ theory. In fact, a history of nineteenth- and twentieth-century medicine could easily read as a history of the achievements of many of humanity's greatest scientific minds.

John Snow's Discovery of Disease Transmission

One such individual was English physician John Snow (1813–1858). Although he was certainly not as prominent as many of his contemporaries, his writings and discoveries clearly offered an empirical foundation for germ theory that would guide future generations of medical researchers. In 1849 Snow published an essay entitled *On the Mode of Communication of Cholera*. In that work, he clearly outlined the mechanism by which the dreaded cholera was transmitted in drinking water. His conclusions amounted to a complete repudiation of miasma as a possible causative factor.

In fact, from his earliest days in medicine, Snow had questioned the essentials of miasma theory. While working in 1832 as a physician's apprentice in Newcastle, a mining town in northern England, the nineteen-year-old Snow witnessed an outbreak of cholera that the local medical establishment attributed to miasmic vapors. Convinced that the disease was not transmitted by air, he noted that "there are a number of facts that have been thought to oppose this evidence: Numerous persons [communicate] with the sick without being affected, and a great number [contract] the disease who have no apparent connection with other patients."[1]

The precocious young apprentice then went on to study the digestive tract of some of the deceased victims of the outbreak, noting that there was a "local [infection] of the mucous membrane of the alimentary canal [the entire digestive tract from mouth to anus]." Based on his examination he concluded that

> the disease must be something which passes
> from the mucous membrane of the alimen-
> tary canal of one patient to that of another,
> which it can only do by being swallowed;
> and as the disease grows in a community by
> what it feeds upon, attacking a few people
> in a town at first, and then becoming more
> prevalent, it is clear that the cholera poison
> must multiply itself by a kind of growth . . .
> taking place in the alimentary canal.[2]

Following an outbreak of cholera in 1854 in London's Soho district, Snow published a second article containing additional evidence in support of his theory that the ailment spreads by ingestion, not by the inhalation of toxic air particles. He reached his conclusion after interviewing many Soho residents. The interviews pointed him in the direction of the source of the infection—a water pump located on London's Broad Street that delivered water to residents of the district. Snow later created a dot map of the entire area hit by the epidemic and was able to illustrate overwhelmingly that the largest number of cases occurred in homes supplied by the Broad Street pump. It was through Snow's efforts that the Broad Street pump was eventually shut down, resulting in a dramatic drop in cholera cases in the area.

However, after repeated attempts at microscopic and chemical examination of the water emitted by the Broad Street pump, Snow was unable to uncover any specific examples of what he had earlier referred to as the cholera poison. The causative agent, a bacterium called *Vibrio cholerae* (sometimes called the "comma bacillus" because of its shape), completely eluded him. Although we do not know whether he and his studies on cholera contributed either directly or even indirectly to the formulation of the germ theory of disease, his professional life and work were indicative of the new turn and radical direction medical science was taking in the nineteenth century.

Laying the Foundation for Preventive Medicine

Most historians of medicine would agree that the magnitude of the discovery of germ theory was shattering in its impact and revolutionary in effect. It necessitated a major recalibration in thinking in the fields of surgery and pathology. And more important, it gave rise to bacteriology, a field of science that deals with microscopic organisms and their relationship to medicine and industrial and agricultural production. Significantly, the individual honored by his peers and successors as the most notable of the medical researchers in this new and indispensable area of modern medicine was the French scientist Louis Pasteur (1822–1895).

By most criteria, Pasteur stands side by side with Isaac Newton (1642–1727), Charles Darwin (1809–1882), and Albert Einstein (1879–1955) as one of the most consequential and influential scientists in history. Pasteur's work laid the foundation for preventive medicine, a new era in medical practice that has resulted in an extension in life expectancy far beyond anything previously experienced or even imagined. But of greater importance, the discoveries he made and therapies he established provided the momentum for the eventual development of wonder drugs such as antibiotics and specific vaccines that would dominate and transform medicine in the twentieth and twenty-first centuries, thereby saving tens of millions of people from premature death. In short, Pasteur made possible a pathway that would eventually lead not only to widespread strides in healing but also to serious studies of human longevity.

Pasteur's most noteworthy and enduring accomplishments derive from his work on immunization. In 1879 an anthrax epidemic broke out in France and other parts of Europe, killing large numbers of sheep and infecting humans as well. Anthrax, an infectious disease caused by a rod-shaped bacterium, *Bacillus anthracis*, attacks both domestic and wild animals. With the patience and thoroughness that had always characterized his work, Pasteur isolated the causative bacillus and discovered that when exposed to air, it lost most of its virulence. (Like many other germs, *Bacillus anthracis* is an anaerobic organism, meaning that it thrives in the absence of free oxygen. When exposed to oxygen, it weakens and eventually dies.) He then developed a vaccine made up of bacilli deliberately exposed to air and therefore considerably less potent.

On May 5, 1881, Pasteur administered the vaccine to twenty-five sheep in a field at Melun, a village south of Paris. A throng of spectators, including local villagers and several members of the French press, watched with great interest. Pasteur carefully left a control group of twenty-five sheep untreated. A few weeks after the initial vaccinations had been completed, on May 31, he took the final, crucial step by administering a fully virulent strain of anthrax to all the sheep, both vaccinated and unvaccinated. Realizing that two or three days would be needed before the results of the experiment could be known, he returned by rail to his home in nearby Paris.

Those momentous results came slightly earlier than Pasteur had anticipated. Early in the morning of June 2, while he was dressing in preparation for his return to Melun, a messenger delivered to him an urgent telegram. Sent by a fellow scientist—one who had consistently rejected Pasteur's theories outright—the message said,

"Stupendous success!"[3] His spirit uplifted by this news, Pasteur took the first train available to Melun. There, as he climbed from the passenger coach, he was surprised to see a crowd of people of all walks of life. Excitedly, they gave him a deafening, prolonged round of applause, and repeated cries of "Miracle! Miracle!"[4] could be heard.

Making his way through the enthusiastic mob, Pasteur soon came to the scene of the experiment, where he saw that twenty-two of the unvaccinated sheep lay dead, while the other three were gravely ill and near death. A few feet away stood the vaccinated animals. All twenty-five were very much alive and well, just as Pasteur had predicted would be the case. Feeling a hand on his shoulder, he turned to see the colleague who had sent the telegram. Once a scientific opponent, he now embraced and congratulated Pasteur and heartily apologized for ever doubting him.

Indeed, this quickly became the typical reaction of the scientific community in general. Pasteur received enthusiastic compliments and approval from most of his peers for his bold and innovative approach to the killer anthrax. Amid such adulation, Pasteur considered that, although English country doctor Edward Jenner (1749–1823) had successfully developed a vaccine for smallpox nearly a century earlier, Jenner had never fully understood the underlying principle that ensured the vaccine's success. Nor had he realized what was responsible for the disease itself, the variola virus. Pasteur, on the other hand, had managed to identify the organism involved (*Bacillus anthracis*) and discovered a method with which to effectively weaken that organism. More importantly, he recognized that the immune systems of humans and animals can build up immunity to a lethal organism when infected earlier by a carefully measured and weakened version of that germ. It was the weakened anthrax germ that Pasteur had effectively utilized as the core of the vaccine itself. A champion of the germ theory of disease, Pasteur's tireless advocacy of it bore fruit, as he is universally regarded as one of the chief scientists most responsible for its eventual acceptance.

Lister and Koch: Pioneers of Antiseptics

Finally, Pasteur possessed an unusual aptitude for articulating his ideas with credibility and clarity. That quality resonated with others, many of whom would join him on medicine's honor roll of eminent research-ers. Two of these scientists, Joseph Lister (1827–1912) and Robert Koch (1843–1910), both contemporaries of Pasteur, are worth recognizing. Lister, a British surgeon, learned of Pasteur's work in the early 1860s. Being a surgeon, he was painfully aware of the fact that it was common for more than 50 percent of all surgical patients to develop fatal infections at the site of their surgical wounds. Lister correctly deduced that airborne microbes successfully entering the wound during the surgical procedure most likely were the culprits.

With that in mind, in 1864 at a hospital in Glasgow, Scotland, Lister started employing carbolic acid, which he reasoned would work as a germ-killing antiseptic, in his operations. He soaked a cloth with the antiseptic and rubbed it on wounds caused by bone fractures. Testing this procedure for a full year, he was thrilled to find that the normal incidence of gas gangrene, a serious infection that often caused patients to die, dropped from 50 percent to only 10 percent. Thereafter, Lister created an apparatus that released a mist containing carbolic acid. With that, he periodically sprayed all the hospital's operating rooms. Not long afterward, he introduced strict rules that mandated sterilizing linens and medical instruments to kill whatever germs they carried. A very professional and fair-minded individual, Lister never failed to partially credit his antiseptic procedures to Pasteur's observation that germs were to be found everywhere— on the ground, in the air, and on and inside the human body.

Meanwhile, Robert Koch, a German physician and researcher who is often referred to as the father of bacteriology, carried Lister's efforts further still. He discovered that using steam to sterilize surgical instruments along with the carbolic acid spray would further reduce the risk of infecting surgical wounds. Among his numerous accomplishments, in 1882 Koch discovered and described the tuberculosis bacterium, for which he was awarded the Nobel Prize in Physiology or Medicine in 1905. In the late nineteenth century, tuberculosis was responsible for the deaths of one out of every seven people living in the United States and Europe. Koch's discovery helped contribute to the effective treatment and control of the deadly bacterium.

Another important contribution Koch made to the fast-expanding field of medical science was a set of four postulates, or basic facts assumed to be true most of the time, regarding germs and disease. They became known as Koch's postulates in his honor. These statements encompass the fundamental experimental method by which one can demonstrate that a given disease has been caused by a specific germ. The four postulates are:

1. The causative agent [of the disease being studied] must be present in every case of the disease and must not be present in healthy animals.

2. The pathogen [disease-causing agent] must be isolated from the diseased host animal and must be grown in pure culture [in a container in the lab].

3. The same disease must be produced when microbes from the pure culture are inoculated [injected] into healthy suscepti-ble animals.

4. The same pathogen must be recoverable once again from this artificially infected host animal, and it must be able to be grown again in pure culture.[5]

Although a few minor exceptions to these basic general rules were found in the succeeding century, they are still an accepted cornerstone of the field of microbiology.

Global Increases in Life Expectancy

Thanks to the work of scientists like Snow, Pasteur, Lister, Koch, and several others, medical science was providing humanity with good reason to view the future hopefully, at least where health and disease were concerned. Indeed, over time an unparalleled increase in average life expectancy and the world's population validated the optimism handed down to the twentieth century by these earlier pioneers in modern medicine. Six thousand years ago, when the first civilizations appeared in the ancient Near East and life expectancy was believed to be around thirty years old, the population of the world stood at approximately 8 million to 10 million. That figure rose in very small increments over the next fifty-five hundred or so years, and by the year 1700, the worldwide population had reached a half billion. It was then that the global population began an unprecedented exponential climb. According to figures compiled by the US Census Bureau, by 1800 that number had nearly doubled as it rose to 900 million. It then continued its ascent and more than doubled to over 2 billion by 1930. Moreover, in the less than a century that followed, by 2022 it had quadrupled to 8 billion. Several factors have contributed to these substantial increases in the human population during the past two hundred years. They include a rapid growth in agricultural output; a series of technological innovations, such as sanitized human waste disposal and water filtration systems; recognition of the importance of educating the public in the essentials of personal hygiene; and the Industrial Revolution and its many related developments and events.

The population growth of the nineteenth and twentieth centuries was also fueled by more than a doubling of the global average life expectancy. In 1800 the global average life expectancy was twenty-eight years. By 2019 it was seventy-three years. The factor that has had arguably the largest impact on this unprecedented increase in global life expectancy has been discoveries and advances in medicine, driven primarily by the widespread acceptance of

Global Life Expectancy, 1770–2019

With the discovery and acceptance of germ theory and the development of vaccines and antibiotics, life expectancy rose sharply starting near the end of the 1800s and continuing into the 2000s.

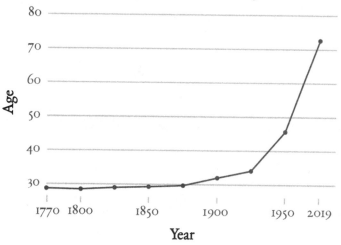

Source: "Life Expectancy, 1770 to 2019," Our World in Data. https://ourworldindata.org.

germ theory. More specifically, twentieth-century medicine's greatest successes have been in dealing with infectious diseases and can be credited to the development and widespread use of vaccines and antibiotic therapy. Both have been responsible for enhancing the physical well-being and longevity of humans throughout the globe, especially in the world's leading industrialized nations, where the economic systems are strong, the political systems are stable, and the health care and educational systems are ubiquitous.

In the United States, for example, the Centers for Disease Control and Prevention (CDC) reports that the twentieth century witnessed dramatic declines in mortality rates (the frequency with which a disease kills sectors of the population) for numerous diseases, especially those for which the vaccination of children was widely employed. During that pivotal century, infections like smallpox, tetanus, and polio experienced a nearly 100 percent decline in death rates in individuals who were immunized. According to the CDC:

> Deaths from infectious diseases declined markedly in the United States during the 20th century. This decline contributed to a sharp drop in infant and child mortality and to the 29.2-year increase in life expectancy. In 1900, 30.4% of all deaths occurred among children aged less than 5 years; [in contrast,] in 1997, that percentage was only 1.4%. In 1900, the three leading causes of death were pneumonia, tuberculosis (TB), and diarrhea and enteritis, which (together with diphtheria) caused one third of all deaths. Of these deaths, 40% were among children aged less than 5 years.... Public health action to control infectious diseases in the 20th century was based on the 19th century discovery of microorganisms as the cause of many serious diseases; [and] dis-

ease control resulted from improvements in sanitation and hygiene, the discovery of antibiotics, and the implementation of universal childhood vaccination programs.[6]

Antibiotics Usher in a New Age of Medicine

Amid all this amazing medical progress in the twentieth century, if one had to pinpoint a single overriding factor that not only saved seemingly countless lives but also contributed to a sharp increase in human life expectancy (at least in developed countries like the United States), one might well choose the introduction of penicillin and other antibiotics. The era of antibiotic therapy began in 1928 when a Scottish bacteriologist, Alexander Fleming (1881–1955), discovered what the world justifiably heralded as *the* miracle drug of the modern age, penicillin. He published his findings the following year, but it would be more than a decade later, during World War II (1939–1945), that the drug was certified for general use. The results of penicillin's role in the war itself were remarkable. Doctors treating the wounded in field hospitals were able to eliminate most infections resulting from battle injuries. In fact, since the amount of penicillin available was limited in the early 1940s, military doctors opted to collect the urine of patients who were on the drug, crystallize the excreted penicillin, and then reuse it.

By 1950 penicillin was being widely distributed for use by the public at large. Considered jointly with vaccines, which were also being used extensively, its efficacy as a way not only to heal but also to extend people's life spans was attested to by demographic figures calculated by the US Census Bureau. In 1800 life expectancy in America was 40 years. By 1900 that figure stood at 46.2 years. And by 2000 life expectancy had leaped to 76.9 years, an unprecedented 66 percent increase in a single century.

Shortly after the war, in 1945, Fleming received the Nobel Prize in Physiology or Medicine. That award was well deserved because penicillin ushered in a new era in contemporary medicine. William Bynum, professor emeritus in the history of medicine at University College London, refers to the period following World War II as the "golden age of modern medicine." He notes that "doctors enjoyed an unprecedented era of prestige and trust. Infectious diseases were believed to be more or less conquered."[7] Even the US Department of Health, Education, and Welfare (HEW), after conferring with various medical specialists throughout the country, declared in 1960 that "[humanity's] mastery over nature has been vastly extended including [its] capacity to cope with diseases and other threats to human life and health."[8] And Dr. William H. Stewart, US surgeon general from 1965 to 1969, echoed the enthusiasm of his HEW colleagues. Once, at a White House gathering of state health officers, he announced that infectious diseases were becoming a negligible problem thanks to medicine's extraordinary success in suppressing them. He opined that public funds could now be diverted from communicable to chronic diseases, proclaiming, "It is time to close the book on infectious diseases and declare the war against pestilence won."[9]

But Stewart's pronouncement proved premature and overly optimistic, as a spate of new bacterial infections that were unresponsive to penicillin therapy began surfacing. Perhaps one of the most plausible explanations for this turn of events may be attributed to the Darwinian concept of natural selection, or survival of the fittest. The concept is quite simple: a random mutation or alteration in the genetic structure of a bacterium could render it immune to an antibiotic that was developed and programmed to ward off that bacterium. In other words, the mutation would compromise the efficacy of the penicillin. Consequently, a colony of mutated bacteria would stand a better chance of surviving a dosage of penicillin than a colony that had never mutated. This situation necessitated the expansion of additional types and classes of antibiotics.

The expanded development of antibiotics peaked during the 1970s. Since then, no new classes of antibiotics have been created, with the search for new antibiotics being replaced by the modification of existing ones.

While more than one hundred antibiotics have been developed and approved since Alexander Fleming's historic discovery, penicillin remains the most widely prescribed antibiotic in the world. As with bacteria, mutations in the composition of viral genes could significantly alter a virus's virulence or power to infect. Biologically, the foremost difference between viruses and bacteria is that bacteria are living cells that can survive both inside or outside a body; viruses are a nonliving collection of molecules that essentially hijack and latch onto a host cell. Since they are not complete cells, once they have invaded and become part of a colony of normal, living cells, they use those cells to reproduce and multiply. While both viruses and bacteria can be developed into effective vaccines, antibiotics are only effective when targeting bacteria.

Today's Medicine in the Global North and South

Due to the herculean efforts of Bacon, Vesalius, Van Leeuwenhoek, Snow, Pasteur, Lister, Koch, Fleming, and other great medical pioneers of the past, the medicine of today has carried humanity across a perilous threshold dominated heretofore by an anonymous and deadly enemy commonly known as disease germs. Most (though regrettably not all) of those troublesome microbes are kept at bay with selective medications and vaccines, while many have been all but eliminated as a serious threat.

This is especially true of the state of medicine in the Global North (developed nations of the world), where chronic illnesses such as cardiovascular disease have replaced communicable disease in claiming the largest number of lives annually.

While it is true that the medicine of today has seen important life-saving advancements in areas of medicine outside infectious disease (cardiology, pulmonology, nephrology), it is the discovery of germs and antimicrobials that have played the biggest role in extending human life expectancy up to this point. As noted in a 2016 article in the journal *Annals of Ibadan Postgraduate Medicine*:

> The antibiotic era revolutionized the treatment of infectious diseases worldwide, although with much success in developed countries. In the US for example, the leading causes of death changed from communicable diseases to non-communicable diseases (cardiovascular disease, cancer, and stroke), the average life expectancy at birth rose to 78.8 years and older population changed from 4% to 13% of the entire US population.[10]

These figures illustrate this connection between victories over communicable diseases and increases in human longevity. They also underscore how and why the medicine of tomorrow will likely focus more on chronic disease management, partly in hopes of helping people live longer, healthier lives.

While the Global North begins to tackle the new leading causes of death (heart disease, cancer, and so forth), many of the emergent nations of the world are still mired in the trenches of germ warfare. Although life expectancy in the Global South (the nations of the developing world) has increased in recent years, that increase does not match comparable statistics in the industrialized world. Given this situation, many residing in the large urban areas of the world's developing countries are not living long enough to die of cardiovascular disease, cancer, or stroke. They are still falling prey to communicable diseases at a much higher rate than people are in the Global North.

For example, the Central African Republic, the developing nation with the lowest life expectancy (forty-eight years), is in that respect on par with the situation that existed globally in 1900 (before antibiotics and the widespread use of vaccines). Unsurprisingly, the leading causes of death in the Central African Republic are all communicable diseases: HIV/AIDS, influenza, and pneumonia. This is a common theme that echoes throughout emergent nations with low life expectancies, and it explains why such regions have the lowest life expectancies in the world. This data also shows that advancements in the area of infectious disease are the true standouts with regard to increasing life expectancy when it comes to discussing the medicine of today.

The problems facing the Global South are multifaceted and ubiquitous. Major socioeconomic issues such as crowded and proliferating slums and urban poverty in those nations are exacerbated by air and water pollution and resource depletion. Politically, many live under the cloud of oppressive governments and are deprived of most, and in some nations all, basic human rights. Malnutrition is common, and a major contributory factor is the spread of most communicable diseases, including tuberculosis, malaria, and HIV/AIDS. In addition, of major significance is the fact that medication and vaccinations, while available in emergent nations, are often not being distributed widely enough; that is, the populations residing in particular areas in many developing countries go unmedicated and unvaccinated.

As we move ahead and examine what possibilities the future of medicine may hold regarding human longevity, we should remind ourselves once again that the "medicine of yesterday" was rife with ignorance and superstition. During the huge outbreak of bubonic plague in Europe and parts of Asia in 1348, for example, humanity knew nothing about its cause or course, yet people had no choice other than to face that disease's awful consequences. Moreover, this so-called Black Death was not discriminatory. When it opened its deadly umbrella of infection, entire nations darkened, and all who resided in them were fair game for the microbes that caused the contagion. No one—not king, nor queen, nor laborer, nor priest—was excepted from the ravages of the plague.

Such is not the case as we explore the medicine of today and tomorrow, where there are those who are in a position to benefit greatly from modern medicine along with those who, either by choice or chance, cannot. As Sangeeta Singh-Kurtz, a journalist who investigates human longevity research, points out, in poorer, developing nations in Africa and Asia, most people still struggle to survive large outbreaks of malaria and other diseases that are rarely seen in developed nations like the United States, and life expectancy in those less well-off countries remains far lower than in the richer nations.

For example, she says, "in the US, where the majority of life-extension technology is being developed, a person born in 1950 could expect to live anywhere between 20 to 25 years longer than one born in 1900." In contrast, she asserts, in 2010 in "Nigeria, the African continent's most populous country . . . the average life expectancy . . . was just over 50, a landmark the US had passed 100 years earlier."[11] Because of this inequity, she adds, in 2015 the famous entrepreneur and philanthropist Bill Gates criticized increasing research into human longevity in wealthier nations. "It seems pretty egocentric," he quipped, "while [the world still labors to fight the ravages of] malaria and TB, for rich people to fund things so they can live longer."[12]

This does not mean that such research should stop, Singh-Kurtz states. Indeed, she says, "most scientists would agree that increasing investments in longevity research are not necessarily a detriment to global health."[13] Yet, she and other expert observers caution, when considering the contrasts between the haves and the have-nots, the world should remain aware that we all live in the same global village. To ignore that interconnectedness as we look into what the future holds for the human life span would not only be an unconscionable moral shortcoming, it may very well turn into a recipe for disaster.

Notes

1. Quoted in Dorothy H. Crawford, *Deadly Companions: How Microbes Shaped Our History*. New York: Oxford University Press, 2009, p. 134.

2. Quoted in Crawford, *Deadly Companions*, p. 134.

3. Quoted in Madeleine P. Grant, *Louis Pasteur: Fighting Hero of Science*. New York: McGraw-Hill, 2021, p. 67.

4. Quoted in Grant, *Louis Pasteur*, p. 67.

5. Quoted in Gwendolyn R.W. Burton and Paul G. Engelkirk, *Microbiology for the Health Sciences*. Philadelphia: Lippincott Williams and Wilkins, 2000, p. 15.

6. Centers for Disease Control and Prevention, "Achievements in Public Health, 1900–1999: Control of Infectious Diseases," July 30, 1999. www.cdc.gov.

7. William Bynum, *The History of Medicine: A Very Short Introduction*. New York: Oxford University Press, 2008, p. 120.

8. US Department of Health, Education, and Welfare, *Final Report: United States. Public Health Service. Study Group on Mission and Organization of the Public Health Service*. Washington, DC: HEW, 1960, p. 5.

9. Quoted in David J. Hunter and Harvey V. Fineberg, *Readings in Global Health: Essential Reviews from the New England Journal of Medicine*. New York: Oxford University Press, 2015, p. 36.

10. W.A. Adediji, "The Treasure Called Antibiotics," *Annals of Ibadan Postgraduate Medicine*, December 14, 2016, pp. 56–57.

11. Sangeeta Singh-Kurtz, "Bill Gates Calls Silicon Valley's Pursuit of Immortality 'Egocentric.' Maybe He's Right," Quartz, March 27, 2019. https://qz.com.

12. Quoted in Paul Tullis, "Are You Rich Enough to Live Forever?," *Town & Country*, March 30, 2017. www.townandcountrymag.com.

13. Singh-Kurtz, "Bill Gates Calls Silicon Valley's Pursuit of Immortality 'Egocentric.'"

Part II

Chapter Three

The Medicine of Tomorrow

Modern medicine—a broad term that describes the evidence-based diagnostics and therapeutics used to alleviate chronic diseases, cure molecular deficiencies, and correct physical conditions—has aided in increasing human life expectancy. However, it is the medicine of tomorrow—being researched today—that will push the average human life span to greater lengths. It should be noted that the terms *life expectancy* and *life span* differ for those in the medical field.

For example, in the United States the average life expectancy—how long a typical individual is expected to live—was 78.6 years in 2021. Life expectancy takes into account genetics, lifestyle, and other factors that commonly influence mortality. On the other hand, life span refers to the maximum number of years humans can live before essential body organs and systems begin to irreparably fail. Currently, the human life span falls somewhere between 120 and 130 years (with some researchers convinced that 150 years might be a possible natural upper limit in age). The oldest human reliably recorded in modern times, a French woman named Jeanne Louise Calment, died in August 1997. Born in 1875, a little more than a year before General George Armstrong Custer (1839–1876) was defeated by a united army of Native Americans near the Little Bighorn River in the Montana Territory, she lived an impressive 122 years and 5 months.

No one knows why Calment lived so long. However, most health professionals believe that people would live longer if they chose healthier diets and lifestyles and if some of the medical obstacles they faced—including limited access to care and the health problems incurred through disease and genetic illness—were removed. A study conducted in 2018 by a team of researchers at Harvard's T.H. Chan School of Public Health found that when a person assumes consistently healthy habits, including eating mostly plant-based foods, exercising regularly, refraining from smoking, and maintaining a healthy body weight—increased life expectancy ensues. The increase, the researchers found, can amount to at least fourteen years for women and twelve years for men.

Attempts to Extend "Health Span"

It is not just the number of extra years that is crucial in such an increase in life expectancy, explains Dr. Frank Hu, director of the Department of Nutrition at the Chan School; it is also important to consider "improving quality of life and reducing overall health care costs."

Extending life span is not enough, he adds. Scientists also "want to extend 'health span,' so that [the span of] a longer life . . . is healthy and free of major chronic diseases and disabilities associated with those diseases."[1]

All the medical advances discussed in the previous two chapters—both individually and cumulatively—have had a considerable impact on improving life expectancy. However, even with those discoveries, the average human living in the industrialized world is still expected to die somewhere around 78.6 years, a little over half the theoretically projected natural limit of the human life span. Until the twenty-first century, the question of extending human life beyond 130 years, and certainly 150 years, remained doubtful. Although the life span of species across the animal kingdom appears ingrained and unchangeable, advancements in science are proving that human longevity can be extended. Thus, the medicine of the future is unique in several respects. It is probable that some of the therapies described as the "medicine of tomorrow" will not only close the gap between life expectancy and life span, a few might even push humanity beyond the theoretical boundaries. This is the medicine with the potential to allow humans eventually to live for more than 150 years, and some within the community of researchers and theoreticians studying human longevity believe that there will be ways to allow people to live hundreds or thousands of years, or perhaps even longer.

Not all longevity experts agree with that assessment, but they readily admit that even if modern medicine can never hope to produce such wondrous outcomes, scientific investigation of aging and human longevity is currently developing at an ever-increasing pace, and predicting what it will lead to is difficult at best. As popular science writer Ferris Jabr summarizes it:

> [As] science discovers increasingly promising ways to slow or reverse aging in the lab, the question of human longevity's potential limits is more urgent than ever. When their work is examined closely, it's clear that longevity scientists hold a wide range of nuanced perspectives on the future of humanity. Historically . . . their outlooks have been divided into two broad camps, which some journalists and researchers call the pessimists and the optimists. Those in the first group view life span as a candle wick that can burn for only so long. They generally think that we are rapidly approaching, or have already reached, a ceiling on life span. . . . In contrast, the optimists see life span as a supremely, maybe even infinitely elastic band. They anticipate considerable gains in life expectancy around the world,

increasing numbers of extraordinarily long-lived people, and eventually supercentenarians [people who reach and surpass the age of 110] who . . . [push] the record to 125, 150, 200 and beyond. Though unresolved, the long-running debate has already inspired a much deeper understanding of what defines and constrains life span and of the interventions that may one day significantly extend it.[2]

Unveiling Diseases' Causes at the Molecular Level

Whether the longevity scientists are so-called pessimists or optimists, the technologies they are exploring at present are in many ways preliminary in nature because few have yet undergone enough scientific scrutiny to be accepted into the mainstream of clinical medical treatment. The fact is that science can sometimes move slowly, especially when it comes to clinical medicine and its use in treating patients. Before new technological concepts and practices can be accepted into common treatment regimens, the benefits must clearly show themselves to outweigh the risks as determined through carefully designed laboratory and clinical trials, many of which can take years to complete. Thus, because many of the technologies introduced in these chapters are still being researched or exist only as theories, it is important to understand that such explorations in and of themselves cannot and do not serve as substitutes for professional medical care.

In addition to not yet being commonly used in everyday clinical medicine, the medicine of tomorrow is deeply rooted in the understanding of molecular mechanisms, especially those involving genetics. It seems as if science and medicine are progressing in a way that continually reveals smaller and smaller aspects of biology—from the macroscopic discovery of the circulatory system to the microscopic discovery of cells to the molecular discovery of DNA. This scientific progression into smaller and smaller spatial realms has led to the unveiling of the true causes of disease at the molecular level. And with the molecular tools now available, scientists can begin to target the source of some diseases. That which cannot be seen with the naked eye may appear mysterious or even intimidating to some, but to know the basic science behind the newly developing technologies, even in their simplest form, will enhance the understanding of their effect on longevity.

Therefore, a foundational understanding of genetics is important to developing a deeper appreciation for the medical advancements described in later chapters. In looking at the fundamentals of genetics, to begin with, DNA—which stands for "deoxyribonucleic acid"—is found in the nucleus of the cell and is often described as the brain of the cell. The nucleus holds the information needed for cells to function, and that information is coded in the DNA, which is made up of single molecules called nucleotides. Many nucleotides strung together in a long chain make up DNA. Although there are only four nucleotides (abbreviated A, T, G, and C), the order in which they are strung together to create DNA allows for numerous possible combinations. And the order of these nucleotides is part of the genetic code. DNA is, on its simplest level, the data that program a cell and tell it how to function by defining which proteins it will make. Proteins are molecules that are often described as the workforce of the cell. Different types of cells require different types of proteins to accomplish the unique functions of that cell.

The genetic code is also made up of numerous genes. A gene is a segment of DNA that codes a specific protein. Every cell in the human body has the same DNA, which means every cell has the same genetic code. At first glance, there might seem to be a problem with that concept. Namely, our skin does not look like our liver, and our brain does not behave like our immune cells; so how can the body have different cell types despite having the same genetic code in each? The answer is that cells are capable of expressing only certain genes while limiting the expression of others. There are an estimated twenty-five thousand genes in the human genome, so there are many combinations of gene expression and silencing that determine what bodily feature or activity each cell is suited to. The genes that skin cells express are going to be different than the genes that liver cells express, which explains why they look different and have different functions. Because they express different genes, they will make different proteins.

This microscopic genetic system can become amazingly complex because the body has over 2 million protein configurations, some only subtly different than others of their type, all coded by the twenty-five thousand genes with distinct functions. The proteins produced help define what the function of each cell is, and that production chain is determined by the genetic machinery reading and either "turning on" or "turning off" specific genes within the DNA. Experts in genetics call that process of reading the genes and turning them on or off "expression."

Epigenetics: Roles of Behavior and the Environment

An entire subdivision of genetic research has developed around the process of expression that does not reflect the genetic sequence. Called epigenetics, it is defined as the study of how human behaviors and the environment in which humans live can cause changes that affect the way the genes work. Because epigenetic changes are influenced by how an individual's body reads a DNA sequence, and also because the genetic machinery can turn genes on or off depending on what it reads, those changes are flexible and reversible. Thus, epigenetic changes occur in response to a person's behaviors, environment, and personal physical characteristics at a given time.

Many overt behaviors can cause measurable epigenetic changes. The CDC cites as an example the somewhat common behavior of smoking, saying that it can cause a reduction in a healthy molecular process known as methylation, in which certain atoms work to repair microscopic damage to one's DNA. The CDC explains:

> At certain parts of the AHRR gene, smokers tend to have less DNA methylation than non-smokers. The difference is greater for heavy smokers and long-term smokers. After quitting smoking, former smokers can begin to have increased DNA methylation at this gene. Eventually, they can reach levels similar to those of non-smokers. In some cases, this can happen in under a year, but the length of time depends on how long and how much someone smoked before quitting.[3]

Other behavioral factors that cause epigenetic changes include exercise, diet (and in a related vein, obesity), drinking alcohol, taking recreational drugs, and sleeping too little. Among the common environmental factors that affect genetic expression are air pollution, heavy metals or various toxic chemicals in the water, excess radiation, and mental stress. Of special interest to the topic of human longevity, in addition to the behavioral and environmental factors already mentioned, simply growing older can cause epigenetic changes.

Indeed, alterations in DNA are affected by the duration of exposure to those diverse factors; that is, the longer one is exposed to certain factors, the more pronounced the epigenetic changes can become. That is why such changes occur as people age, and carefully measuring such changes on a microscopic level can reveal a person's approximate age, similar to how rings on the inside of a tree can demonstrate the tree's age and mark where it encountered unusual levels of damage or stress.

Exploring such epigenetic changes in increasing detail is only one of the technological approaches that longevity scientists have been employing in recent years in their ongoing attempt to discover ways of prolonging human life. But to date it is also without question one of the most promising. This was shown when in early 2022 scientists at the Salk Institute for Biological Studies in La Jolla, California, announced a breakthrough in slowing the aging process. A spokesperson for the facility described how Salk researchers had used epigenetic technology on mice. In layman's terms, the scientists injected what they called "reprogramming molecules," known as Yamanaka factors (discussed later), into key cells in the test animals.

The noteworthy results were that this procedure reset the epigenetic system of the mice to the way it had been when they were younger. "When the researchers looked at normal signs of aging in the animals that had undergone the treatment," the spokesperson says,

> they found that the mice, in many ways, resembled younger animals. In both the kidneys and skin, the epigenetics of treated animals more closely resembled epigenetic patterns seen in younger animals. When injured, the skin cells of treated animals had a greater ability to proliferate and were less likely to form permanent scars. Older animals usually show less skin cell proliferation and more scarring. Moreover, metabolic molecules in the blood of treated animals did not show normal age-related changes.[4]

The importance of this study was clear. Employing epigenetic technology, researchers had succeeded in not just slowing down the aging process in test mice; rather, it appeared that they had reversed it, even if to only a small degree. "At the end of the day," remarks Pradeep Reddy, one of the study's directors, "we want to bring resilience and function back to older cells so that they are more resistant to stress, injury and disease. This study shows that, at least in mice, there's a path forward to achieving that."[5] This achievement was not lost on other human longevity researchers around the globe, for they understood that often in science new therapies that work in test animals are eventually applicable to human beings. These researchers anticipate that the success of such experiments indicates that the aging process and its impact on the human body might be tempered with technology and that the body might remain more resilient as human life span increases.

Notes

1. Quoted in Alice Park, "Scientists Calculated How Much Longer You Can Live with a Healthy Lifestyle," *Time*, June 8, 2020. https://time.com.

2. Ferris Jabr, "How Long Can We Live?," *New York Times*, October 1, 2021. www.nytimes.com.

3. Centers for Disease Control and Prevention, "What Is Epigenetics?," August 15, 2022. www.cdc.gov.

4. Quoted in Salk Institute for Biological Studies, "Cellular Rejuvenation Therapy Safely Reverses Signs of Aging in Mice," March 7, 2022. www.salk.edu.

5. Quoted in Salk Institute for Biological Studies, "Cellular Rejuvenation Therapy Safely Reverses Signs of Aging in Mice."

Chapter Four

Regenerative Medicine

Unfortunately for humanity, every day various natural and artificial elements work against people's health and longevity. For instance, human cells and organs are regularly bombarded with various substances that can damage tissues and impair the functioning of organ systems. High blood sugar destroys kidney tissue; consumption of drugs and alcohol destroys liver tissue; and inhalation of pollutants such as cigarette smoke destroys lung tissue. Even diseases beyond people's control that arise without warning can impair the health of bodily organs. Consequently, over time human organs degenerate or lose their capacity to function as the cells within them die off. When the degeneration is severe enough, organ failure may occur. Organ failure is a commonplace occurrence, as evidenced by the large number of patients with end-stage renal disease, cirrhosis of the liver, and fibrosis of the lungs—many of them awaiting transplants for new and healthy organs. The unfortunate reality is that far too many of those individuals die before an organ transplant becomes available, even if they are lucky enough to make it onto the organ transplantation list. Clearly, these and similar adverse health issues work against the concept of helping humans live longer.

This is where the field of regenerative medicine enters the picture. This field can not only save people's lives but possibly—in the near future—extend the average length of those lives. In the words of Dr. Michael West, noted pioneer researcher in the fields of stem cells and cellular aging:

> I would define regenerative medicine as
> that collection of technologies that utilizes
> . . . [certain bodily cells with specialized
> functions] to regenerate tissues in the body
> ravaged from disease, primarily degenera-
> tive disorders associated with aging. . . . If
> we can learn the lessons of how our repro-
> ductive lineage has been creating babies for
> millions of years to continue the human
> species, we should be able to design med-
> ical therapies to allow the human body
> to regenerate itself and escape the genetic
> boundaries of human life.[1]

Filling the Hole Created by an Injury

Before examining what regenerative medicine is and how it may one day add years to human life spans, it is necessary to clarify two important related concepts—repair and regeneration. When human bodily tissues in an organ are injured, the cells that make up those tissues die, leaving the organ with what amounts to a hole to fill. The organ essentially has two means of filling in the gap so that it can continue to function—repair or regeneration. As individuals steadily grow older, the delicate balance between tissue repair and regeneration tips in favor of repair due to the natural aging of people's cells.

If the damage is severe or persistent, it is likely that the body will opt to repair it. The repair pathway is essentially a crude patch. The patch serves no physiological function other than preserving the structural integrity of the tissue. This process occurs when repair cells lay down fibrous scar tissue over the damaged area. This scar tissue is simply extracellular protein scaffolding whose sole purpose is to hold the rest of the tissue together. The drawback of this is that the individual will lose some organ functionality because the organ has lost some functional tissue.

In contrast, the second possible way to fill the hole created by the injury—the regenerative pathway—involves the proliferation of new, specialized cells to replace damaged ones and rebuild tissue. In this process, those specialized cells fill in the afflicted area. In comparison to fibrous scar tissue, these cells can perform the same functions of the cells they are replacing. The degree of success of the procedure depends on the number and health of the specialized cells present in the tissue that was damaged.

Stem Cells to Replace Diseased Organs

West and other longevity scientists hope that regenerative medicine will be able to replace diseased organs in humans as they age, just as a mechanic replaces old car parts as they break down. According to these experts, there are two general ways to go about regenerating tissue. One is through the work of the specialized cells mentioned earlier, which scientists technically refer to as stem cells. Stem cells are undifferentiated cells that can produce new cells indefinitely. That they are undifferentiated means that they have not yet matured into a specific kind of adult cell, such as heart cell, liver cell, kidney cell, or some other sort of mature cell associated with a specific organ or type of tissue. There are different kinds of stem cells in a human body. One, called pluripotent, consists of cells that are mainly present in developing embryos. They can potentially go on to produce any and every kind of cell in the body. That is, they can produce cells that will eventually form the gastrointestinal tract, the nervous system, the heart, connective tissue (including skin), and so forth. Therefore, pluripotent cells are highly promising for their capacity to regenerate new cells and organs. That includes the provocative prospect of growing replacement tissues and organs outside the body and implanting them in place of damaged versions. Such artificially created organs, says Paola Bonfanti, a leading researcher in regenerative medicine,

> have been on the horizon for some years now. They present many challenges but, if we can overcome them, they will open up the possibility for patients who need a new organ no longer having to wait for a human donor. . . . In [the near future] we will see significant breakthroughs around how artificial organs function, while the technology used to produce them will take them one step closer to use in the clinic. To date, the greatest success we have had in this field has been the production of lab-grown epidermis, the outermost layer of skin, to replace that which has been destroyed by burns. This is achieved by growing the stem cells of a patient's own epidermis (from an area spared by the burn) in culture and then transferring [the new cells] to . . . the af-

fected [skin] surface. The new epidermis at-
taches and functions for decades, although
it is unable to produce hair or sebaceous
glands. This technique has saved the lives
of thousands of burns patients and is in use
in hospitals across the world.[2]

Indeed, stem cell transplant therapies like the kind
Bonfanti describes are potentially helpful models to
follow in designing methods of regeneration for all the
bodily organs and at the same time holding out hope for
prolonging life through such organ regeneration. The
chief method for such transplants, according to experts,
will be the use of so-called induced pluripotent stem
cells (or iPSCs for short). These are cells that started out
as ordinary, non-pluripotent, undifferentiated cells but
are at some point reprogrammed by the body to become
pluripotent, more specialized cells. Prior to the discovery
of iPSCs, it was assumed that a mature cell could not be
brought back to an undifferentiated state. That is, it was
believed that a mature liver cell was unable to become an
adult liver stem cell and that an adult liver stem cell was
unable to go back to being a pluripotent stem cell. Once
the pluripotent stem cells of the embryo developed into
mature stem cells in the adult, there was supposedly no
going back to pluripotency. Thus, it was thought that

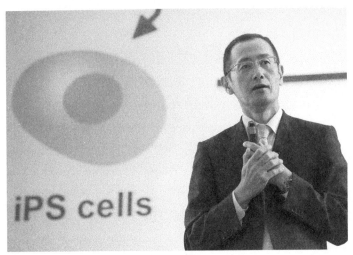

In 2006, Dr. Shinya Yamanaka, seen here speaking at an event in 2012, discovered that it is possible to induce pluripotency in a cell.

skin stem cells could only produce skin cells and that they could not suddenly become small bowel stem cells.

This widely held belief was proved incorrect thanks to the work of Shinya Yamanaka (b. 1962), a researcher affiliated with Japan's Kyoto University. In 2006 his lab made the discovery that it is possible to induce pluripotency in a cell. In other words, he found a way to reset the age of a cell backward essentially to zero. Furthermore, he discovered a means to take any cell in the human body and reprogram it into a pluripotent stem cell. These reprogrammed cells are the iPSCs. The mechanism behind this reprogramming involves the activation of four Yamanaka factors that, when transferred into a mature cell, convince the cell to perform like it did when it was still in the embryo. In a sense, Yamanaka tricked the cell into believing it was back in the womb and therefore should be pluripotent. Such cells reprogram themselves and in essence turn back their age, thereby acquiring much regenerative potential. Yamanaka's work with iPSCs earned him the Nobel Prize in Physiology or Medicine in 2012.

iPSCs and Human Life Expectancy

The award was well deserved because the importance of Yamanaka's discovery cannot be overstated. Its implications will surely contribute to the extension of human life expectancy as, in time, the use of iPSCs likely becomes a mainstay therapy within the realm of regenerative medicine. One such therapeutic potential of iPSCs originates from its ability to differentiate into any cell in the body. Once an iPSC is generated using the four Yamanaka factors, it can be programmed to differentiate into specific tissues found within different organs. This is accomplished by growing the iPSCs in petri dishes next to samples of the cells that scientists want them to become. For example, iPSCs that are grown next to liver cells will develop into liver cells. This forms the basis for regeneration. It is one way in which medicine will be able to replace diseased organs, like replacing old parts of a car, and in the process allow people to live a good deal longer than they normally would have. As West points out:

The good news is that we found a way to identify iPSC cells that have reset the clock of aging. And . . . we've shown [that] it can be made to work quite simply. So the ability to reverse the aging of human cells both from the standpoint of embryological development and in terms of the clock of aging and in an ethically non-problematic manner, and to do it on a commercial and affordable scale, makes regenerative medicine an attractive pathway to profoundly intervene in human aging.[3]

Another therapeutic advantage of iPSCs is that they are constructed from cells that come from the patient's own body (often facilitated by swabbing the inside of the cheek for skin cells). Hence, even when they are being used outside the body to grow a new organ in a lab, they contain the same DNA as the person they came from. Therefore, when such organs are transplanted into that person, they will not be rejected by the immune system as foreign, which commonly happens when someone with different DNA donates an organ to another individual.

A Time Machine of Cell Reprogramming

The medical potential of iPSCs in the realm of regenerative medicine, which in a sense consists of reprogramming cells and organs to work like they did when they were still new, is nothing less than spectacular. West cites only a few of the ways an aging body might be revitalized by such therapies, saying:

> When taken back in this time machine of reprogramming to make all the cell types of the human body pristine, [doctors will have] the ability to regenerate the inner ear for hearing loss in aging, the retina for macular degeneration, part of the midbrain in Parkinson's disease, the heart muscle to deal with the number one killer, heart disease, and cartilage, which has no regenerative capacity whatsoever and whose loss is the number one complaint of the elderly, and so on. By taking the cells back in time, both from an aging standpoint and also by taking them back in time in development to make [younger-acting] cells, we hope to unlock early pathways of embryological development . . . to profoundly regenerate

tissues, such as re-growing amputated limbs and so on.[4]

Incredible advances of this kind will allow the regeneration of tissue in almost any part of the body. They will also make possible the transplantation of newly grown organs and limbs of various kinds into aging bodies, giving their owners what amounts to a new lease on life by letting them live a good deal longer. As an example, West mentions using such iPSC therapies to cure macular degeneration in the eye. In 2022 research in that very area was already in the early phases of clinical trials under the direction of the National Institutes of Health. Another example of a potential application of this technology is in the effort to eradicate muscular dystrophy. Many scientists believe that iPSC therapies will at some point in the near future replace the nonfunctional muscle stem cells responsible for the progressive muscle weakness this disease causes. Even cosmetic conditions such as hair loss due to the death of stem cells in the dermal papillae of hair follicles are being considered for iPSC therapy.

Based on these developments and others like them, there seems to be little doubt that the field of stem cell research will soon find ways of bringing stem cell therapy to clinics worldwide to fight against and hopefully greatly reduce the incidence of ailments such as liver, kidney, and heart failure. If this does come to pass, we will likely see a measurable rise in human life expectancy as fewer patients die from these and other debilitative conditions and diseases that are closely associated with aging.

Bodily Regeneration Through 3-D Printing

Furthermore, there is another area of regenerative medicine that promises to leave its mark on human longevity—bioprinting. In 1984 Charles Hull (b. 1939), an inventor and American engineer, successfully applied for a patent for a copy machine that would hopefully go beyond the kind already in use—that is, the ones that reproduced sheets of paper with printing on them. His version was designed to copy three-dimensional objects. The process was initially called stereolithography. Essentially, Hull succeeded in designing a printer that could print in all three dimensions, guided by computer-aided design programs. The concept was to program a computer to direct the creation of a given object not only very precisely but also in a fraction of the time it would take for it to be otherwise constructed industrially (i.e., by physically shaping, cutting, molding, and fastening the various individual parts into a finished whole).

It did not take long for this new process, popularly known as 3-D printing, to enter the world of medicine and health care. Among the early attempts to use the new technology to aid doctors was that of Belgian researcher Fried Vancraen in 1990. Using an early version of a 3-D printer, he programmed the machine to build up thin layers of a plastic-like material to create an anatomically accurate three-dimensional model of a human skull. Years later Vancraen recalled the way such models were used by surgeons to help plan operations:

> Our first challenge back in the early nineties was to successfully and accurately reproduce human anatomy. Once this was accomplished, 3-D printing already started proving its relevance for very complex operations. Anatomical models were printed that aided in the planning for operations to separate conjoined twins, for complex facial reconstructions, and for treating complicated congenital deformations. . . . [Later, the technology came to be] used by medical device companies, research centers, and hospitals worldwide.[5]

Also during the 1990s and into the early 2000s, other researchers suspected that the 3-D printing process might be employed in regenerative medicine, specifically for printing not just static objects like model skulls but living organs that could replace diseased or injured ones. Among these visionaries was Dr. Anthony Atala of the world-renowned Boston Children's Hospital. He not only kept up with the latest news about ongoing experiments with 3-D printers, in 2004 he also learned about the plight of ten-year-old Luke Massella, whose bladder was failing partly because he had been born with the spinal deformity known as spina bifida. "I was kind of facing the possibility I might have to do dialysis for the rest of my life," Luke later recalled. "I wouldn't be able to play sports, and have the normal kid life."[6]

Atala approached Luke and his mother and told them about recent experiments with 3-D printers. It was a long shot, Atala cautioned, but just maybe he might be able to print the boy a new bladder. When the family agreed it was worth a try, Atala took some cells from the boy's failing bladder, mixed them with various other biological substances, and placed them into a specially modified 3-D printer. In only a few hours the device fashioned what looked and felt like a human bladder; the burning question was whether it would work like a real bladder after being implanted into Luke's body.

The answer to that momentous question came after a historic, marathon operation lasting fourteen grueling hours. The new, completely artificial bladder functioned normally. Moreover, it not only lasted for the year or so that Atala estimated it might if Luke was lucky, it went on working, without a major hitch, year after year. Indeed, following that single surgery, Luke Massella said in an interview in 2019, "Pretty much I was able to live a normal life."[7]

Despite the remarkable success of Atala's transplantation of an artificial bladder, bioprinting of human organs remains largely experimental, in part because in the majority of such transplantation attempts, the patients' bodies have rejected the new organs. Exactly why this happens remains unclear, and surgeons worldwide still marvel that for some inexplicable reason Luke Massella's body did not reject his new bladder. Nevertheless, Atala and other researchers continue to work on this promising technological medical approach, certain that, because it worked perfectly once, it holds great promise once the technique is perfected. Meanwhile, a series of smaller, less complex tissue transplants using 3-D printing have been accomplished with success, including some involving teeth, ears, cartilage, bones, individual blood vessels, and skin.

Although the challenge of perfectly reproducing complex human organs like hearts and kidneys remains elusive, research into bioprinting such organs continues in many countries. Some experts think that within a decade or two, most hospitals will have their own bioprinters in-house or, at the very least, outsource organ bioprinting for their patients. Jordan Miller, a bioengineer at Rice University in Houston, Texas, states:

We're seeing an acceleration in how bio-printing is influencing the field of regenerative medicine. . . . I believe the innovation in materials, and printing technologies will play a pivotal role in what is accomplished in the [near future]. . . . The advancements in and availability of these solutions are yielding a rapid increase in the number of papers published as the technology becomes easier to use, helping the entire regenerative medicine community get closer to our goal of implantable human tissues and organs.[8]

Increasing Longevity No Longer Science Fiction

If Miller's predictions turn out to be accurate, at that point bioprinting will almost certainly have the capability to help extend human life, especially for those who otherwise might perish for lack of a transplanted organ. Furthermore, regenerative medicine in general, including both bioprinting and using stem cell technology to grow organs in a lab, may extend human life expectancy further than many people today conceive. Among the scientists who are hopeful that such increases in longevity will take place is Michael West. "The world of health-span and longevity is no longer science fiction," he declares, and one of the great engines that is going to move the field forward is regenerative medicine. The combination of cell-based therapies with the convergence of technologies that we now have, and the perception that aging is the common factor of so many chronic diseases—it's all coming together. . . . This is going to change medicine. In the end, cell-based therapies are going to be curative, and represent a huge shift in medicine and human health. We are in uncharted territory, and I am absolutely thrilled and agog at what this convergence of technology means and its implications.[9]

Notes

1. Quoted in Gregory M. Fahy and Saul Kent, "Immortal Stem Cells for Anti-Aging Therapies," *Life Extension Magazine*, January 2021. www.lifeextension.com.

2. Paola Bonfanti, "Lab-Grown Organs Could Solve the Transplant Crisis," *Wired*, December 17, 2020. www.wired.co.uk.

3. Quoted in Fahy and Kent, "Immortal Stem Cells for Anti-Aging Therapies."

4. Quoted in Fahy and Kent, "Immortal Stem Cells for Anti-Aging Therapies."

5. Quoted in Tiger Buford, "6 Questions with Fried Vancraen, a Pioneer Who Is Reshaping the Future of Orthopedics with 3D Printing," OrthoStreams, November 22, 2015. https://orthostreams.com.

6. Quoted in Padraig Belton, "A New Bladder Made from My Cells Gave Me My Life Back," BBC, September 11, 2018. www.bbc.com.

7. Quoted in Belton, "A New Bladder Made from My Cells Gave Me My Life Back."

8. Quoted in Vanesa Listek, "2022 Predictions: Bioprinting Leaders Weigh In," 3DPrint.com, December 28, 2021. https://3dprint.com.

9. Quoted in Fahy and Kent, "Immortal Stem Cells for Anti-Aging Therapies."

Chapter Five

Genetic Engineering

The field of genetics made decisive strides in the decades following the discovery of the structure of DNA in 1953. And in 2010 scientists found a link between certain genes and human longevity. This has prompted optimism that genetic research will open doors to increasing the human life span. As science writer Nicholette Zeliadt summarizes it:

> New research suggests that an important indicator of your probable life span may be your genes. Scientists have identified unique genetic signatures strongly associated with a long and healthy life, findings that could help to further the understanding of how certain genes may offer protection from common age-related diseases like cancer, dementia and cardiovascular disease. And one day the data might lead to the development of genetic tests to predict whether a person can expect to live into old

age as well as guide intervention efforts to prevent age-related illness.[1]

To understand how genes might contribute to longer human life spans, it helps to have a precise idea of what genes are. The basic unit of heredity, passed from parent to child, a gene is a small section of the complex chemical DNA. Multiple genes exist in a series, one after another, on long chains of genetic material called chromosomes, which are located inside the nucleus of each cell. About twenty-five thousand genes can be found within a human cell. The genes contain instructions that tell the body to create specific physical characteristics, or traits, including eye color, hair color, height, and so on. And the full set of instructions in the gene constitutes a person's genetic code.

Groundbreaking Experiments in Gene Editing

Once science understood the basics of the human genetic code, researchers took up the challenge of editing it. Gene editing consists of modifying a gene within the DNA of a living thing, whether animal or plant. Some gene editing happens naturally. Scientists first observed this microscopic process in 1987 when studying bacteria. When a virus invaded the bacteria, the latter's DNA underwent changes, including splices, or cuts, that helped destroy the virus if it attacked the bacteria again. The tiny DNA sequences that did the cutting, acting like a microscopic pair of scissors, received the catchy name of CRISPR in 2005. (That acronym stands for "clustered regularly interspaced short palindromic repeats.")

Not surprisingly, researchers around the world wanted to learn to artificially manipulate the CRISPR editing process and convert it into a technology with which they could systematically alter DNA. That goal was achieved in 2011 by chemist and biologist Jennifer Doudna (b. 1964) of the University of California, Berkeley, and Emmanuelle Charpentier (b. 1968), founder and director of the Max Planck Unit for the Science of Pathogens in Berlin, Germany. In 2012 the two published a ground-breaking paper in the journal *Science*, in which they explained how they had learned to control CRISPR's "molecular scissors." The impressive level and precision of their gene-editing technology earned them the Nobel Prize in Chemistry in 2020.

The ability to edit genes is finding application not only in the science of medicine (where it can be used to fight various hereditary diseases and other maladies) but also in the realm of human longevity. This is because doing some highly targeted editing of certain genes seems to hold the promise of making individuals live longer than they would without such editing. Earlier experiments with the genes of some lower life-forms indicate this may well be the case. For example, in recent years researchers in labs worldwide have located genes in fruit flies that are associated with life span. Initial editing of those genes made the flies live about 10 percent longer.

Of course, researchers are aware that physiologically speaking, flies are a far cry from mammals, including humans. What was needed was evidence that editing specific genes in a mammal could result in making that creature live longer. Such evidence was provided in 2021 by scientists at Bar-Ilan University in Ramat Gan, Israel. Working with 250 mice, they noticed that the amount of SIRT6, a protein that aids in naturally occurring repairs to DNA, decreased as the mice aged. The researchers reasoned that if they could reverse that trend, the mice's cells would be healthier and those animals would age less. To

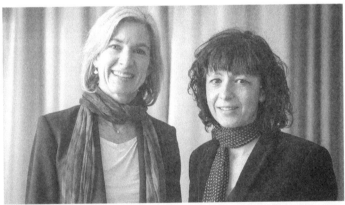

American biochemist Jennifer Doudna (on the left) and French microbiologist Emmanuelle Charpentier (seen here in 2016) were awarded the Nobel Prize in Chemistry in 2020 for developing a highly precise gene-editing technology.

that end, the scientists employed gene editing to increase the supply of SIRT6 in the mice.

The results were dramatic. The mice that received a boost in their SIRT6 lived a whopping 23 percent longer than mice in a control group that did not receive the extra SIRT6. "The change in life expectancy is significant, when you consider that an equivalent jump in human life expectancy would have us living on average until almost 120," states Bar-Ilan University scientist Haim Cohen. Furthermore, Cohen points out, the rejuvenated mice were also livelier, had lower cholesterol, could run faster, and had lower instances of cancer than the control mice. The importance of this study was not lost on the investigators; clearly, they realized, if the life expectancy of one species of mammal could be extended via manipulation of its genes, it was likely that other mammalian species, including humans, could be similarly affected. As Cohen puts it, "The changes we saw in mice may be translatable to humans, and if so that would be exciting."[2]

From that point on, efforts to find human genes that could be edited to help increase longevity intensified. And it did not take long for a breakthrough to materialize. In 2022 a team of researchers in the United Kingdom, co-led by geneticist Nazif Alic of University College London, announced that they had found the particular kind of human genes being sought. Alic writes:

> We have already seen from extensive previous research that inhibiting [via gene editing] certain genes involved in making proteins in our cells, can extend lifespan in model organisms such as yeast, worms and flies. . . . Here, we have found that inhibiting these genes may also increase longevity in people, perhaps because they are most useful early in life before causing problems in late life.[3]

Will Genetic Methods Slow Down Aging?

It therefore appears highly likely that gene-editing technology and other genetics-related therapies expected to emerge in the next few decades will be instrumental in slowing down the aging process. The degree to which genetic methods will extend life is, of course, currently difficult to predict. However, it is already very clear that no matter what new technology is involved, no magic bullet exists that will allow a scientist or clinic or other agency to extend the life of humanity all at once. Rather, at least when it comes to using gene editing to increase longevity, it must be applied on a case-by-case basis, for different individuals have different ailments, genetic predisposi-tions, or other circumstances that may be inhibiting their potential longevity. Each person will need to be evaluated and then agree to the procedure before receiving a target-ed therapy. Given those constraints, such therapies will, at least for the foreseeable future, benefit one person at a time and not be an antiaging panacea for humanity as a whole.

These experiments are exciting and seem to offer some people alive today the possibility that their lives might be extended by not merely a few years but in some cases as many as twenty, thirty, or even sixty or more years, depending on how old they are when they receive the therapy. This promise will squarely impact those indi-viduals who suffer from genetic disorders, conditions like sickle-cell anemia and cystic fibrosis. Many of those ailments can and often do cause premature death in suf-ferers (sometimes as early as age fifteen), who might have far longer lives if they undergo CRISPR editing that can edit out defects in the genetic code.

Indeed, although the technology has not been entirely perfected, it has already been used on a few individuals with genetic disorders. The first patient to benefit was Victoria Gray of Forest, Mississippi. She was only three months old when she first endured an attack of sickle-cell anemia. As the years passed, she increasingly suffered from severe pain and debilitating fatigue, and frequently had to receive blood transfusions. Moreover, by the time she entered her thirties, she could no longer walk or feed herself. Then in 2019 Gray volunteered to be a subject for an experimental gene-editing therapy at the Sarah Cannon Research Institute (SCRI) in Nashville, Tennessee. Longevity researcher Sergey Young picks up the narrative, recalling that

> doctors at the SCRI removed bone marrow from Gray's body and altered the genes of her cells. The procedure effectively "edited" the defect, the way you might go through the lines of a book and correct typos or alter words. The doctors then reintroduced billions of these enhanced cells back into her body to see if they would start doing their job properly. One year after the treatment, Gray appeared to be doing marvelously. While SCRI researchers hoped that at least 20% of Gray's red blood cell system would be positively affected by the procedure, when they checked nine months later, the vast majority of bone marrow cells and hemoglobin proteins found in Gray's body appeared to be functioning effectively. More importantly, her pain attacks and hospital visits had ceased completely![4]

It is hardly surprising that Gray was ecstatic. "I'm doing great," she exclaimed in an interview with NPR in late 2021. "I haven't any problems with sickle cell at all. . . . This is major for me and my family. Two years without me being in the hospital? Wow. We just can't believe it. But we're so grateful."[5]

Meanwhile, the experiment's success made news, and researchers around the world began trying to repeat it with sufferers of various genetic disorders. Close to fifty had undergone gene editing by January 2022; of those, twenty-two, or almost half, had responded positively. Experts see this as extremely promising for ending the suffering of many thousands of people with genetic disorders in the coming years. Furthermore, several of those experts have pointed out that patients who have benefited from the therapy will have their life expectancy increased, possibly dramatically. Gray's doctors are confident that she will live a good deal longer than she would have without the therapy, and the same will be true for the millions of people around the world who will eventually undergo it.

As those individuals receive their therapies on a one-by-one basis, they will eventually mingle with many otherwise healthy people who will, also one by one, seek to extend their lives through genetic engineering. Although most of the members of that second group will likely have always thought of aging as an inevitable reality of life, many will come around to accepting a brave new truth, one that journalist Laurie Mathena has described as "the idea that aging itself is not an inescapable process, but a curable condition."[6]

Notes

1. Nicholette Zeliadt, "Live Long and Proper: Genetic Factors Associated With Increased Longevity Identified," *Scientific American*, July 1, 2010. www.scientificamerican.com.

2. Quoted in Tony Ho Tran, "Scientists Gene Edit Mice to Live 23 Percent Longer," Futurism, June 5, 2021. https://futurism.com.

3. Quoted in Victoria Rees, "Genes Newly Linked to Ageing and Human Lifespan," Drug Target Review, January 26, 2022. www.drugtargetreview.com.

4. Sergey Young, "The Science and Technology of Growing Young," *Life Extension Magazine*, February 1, 2022. www.lifeextension.com.

5. Quoted in Rob Stein, "First Sickle Cell Patient Treated with CRISPR Gene-Editing Still Thriving," NPR, December 31, 2021. www.npr.org.

6. Quoted in Young, "The Science and Technology of Growing Young."

Chapter Six

Antiaging

Every idea, tool, and type of technology so far discussed, including regenerative medicine and genetic engineering, is now contributing, or will in time contribute, to the prolongation of human life expectancy. However, none of them are yet able to augment the natural human life span that appears to be hardwired into the human species. Put another way, these therapies cannot slow or eliminate the aging process itself. At least at present, no amount of stem cell transplants or gene editing can increase the number of years nature has allotted human beings. In short, none of these therapies can offer a cure for what some have called the mother of all diseases—aging.

Gerontologists and others who specialize in geriatric medicine agree that at present, the ability of a human being to recover from life's typical array of illnesses and stress factors continually decreases to the point that the individual simply succumbs to a "natural death." The older we become, the less physiological resilience to the relentless aging process we can expect to muster.

These are the general conclusions of a study published online in late May 2021 in the prestigious journal *Nature Communications*, which closely looked at the medical data of more than five hundred thousand people in the United States, United Kingdom, and Russia. As one expert observer sums up the study's findings:

> [The ultimate] hard limit on human life is 150 years. The main factor limiting our lifespan is a loss of the ability to bounce back after a setback, called "physiological resilience." Even without major health issues, like cancer, your body will eventually run out of energy to help recover from even minor challenges. Even if you somehow manage to make it through decades of old age without a single major health issue—evading cancer, heart disease, diabetes, and so on—scientists say there's a ceiling on how long you can extend your life. . . . But the thing that's keeping the human body from reaching immortality is surprisingly mundane: over time, your body loses the . . . ability to bounce back, [a capacity] that you once had in your younger years.[1]

Some medical researchers and doctors believe that this hardwiring of the aging process can be overcome to one degree or another and based on that bold premise are now looking at ways to bolster the natural resilience of the body in its youth, thereby preventing bodily decline and countering the aging process. They hope that such research, coupled with the various medical technologies that are working toward keeping humans disease free, will not only allow a lot more people to make it into the 120- to 150-year "age club" but possibly enable some individuals to live beyond 150 years. If advances in anti-aging science do come to pass, they will almost literally turn back the clocks of our cells so that, although we may chronologically age, biologically we may retain the appearance and overall good health of a much younger person.

Avoid Waiting Until You Are Sick

This differentiation between chronological and biological age is crucial to the discussion of antiaging. The fact is that there is a significant distinction between those two ways of defining age. Chronological age is what we answer when asked how old we are. It is simply the number of times the earth has carried us around the sun, part of an inexorable cycle that began when the solar system formed more than 4 billion years ago. However, biological age is based on the condition and overall health of a person's cells, tissues, organs, and other body parts, which are blissfully oblivious to the number of times they have made that cosmic journey. Medical researchers point out that determining the biological age of a person is far more personalized and important than simply falling back on conventional chronological age guidelines—ones that suggest that at a given age a person should be expected to show certain signs of aging. After all, some people look and act far younger than some other individuals of the same chronological age.

Apart from lengthening human life span, antiaging research will broadly shift the perspective of medicine. Modern medicine is heavily focused on treating diseases as they emerge. Certainly, there is some preventive medicine that individuals can take advantage of, such as exercising, eating healthy, and getting good sleep. But prevention efforts pale in comparison to medicine's fight against active diseases. For many, a twenty-minute yearly well-check visit with a family doctor is all they get in terms of preventive medicine. Unfortunately, many busy people tend to wait until they are sick before they visit their doctor, which means that their approach to health issues is to react to the onset of illness rather than act to prevent that onset. When something serious happens, doctors strive to reverse the process—that is, bring about a return to normalcy—but that effort is always a reaction after the fact, and doctors agree that patients are better served if they pursue preventive care.

David A. Sinclair (b. 1969), a biologist at Harvard Medical School and a leader in the growing medical field of antiaging, has long cautioned people to avoid the "wait until sick" approach to health and well-being. "Instead of practicing health care in this country," he says, "we're practicing sick care, or what I call 'whack-a-mole' medicine. Medical research is moving towards not just putting Band-Aids on the symptoms of disease, but getting at the major root cause of all major diseases, which is aging itself." In fact, Sinclair is one of the growing number of researchers who see aging as much more than a natural process biologically built into the human species. Rather than being inevitable, he states confidently, aging is very likely treatable. Granted, he adds, "people don't [normally] think about aging as something that is treatable or should be treated like a disease. But it *is* a disease. It's just a very common one."[2]

According to Sinclair and other longevity researchers, as it develops, antiaging therapy will shift medicine from being reactive to proactive. Instead of waiting for diseases and conditions heavily associated with aging, such as diabetes, heart attacks, or dementia to impair health, antiaging therapy has the potential to prevent them from occurring in the first place. In this view, if such therapy induced all the cells in a person's body to look and act like cells from a twenty-five-year-old, then, despite aging chronologically, that individual might be able to retain the biological age of twenty-five for many years and in so doing avoid diseases or other damaging health events associated with aging. Dr. Nir Barzilai (b. 1955), founding director of the Institute for Aging Research at Albert Einstein College of Medicine, thinks that such a scenario, though now seemingly in the realm of science fiction, will be possible in the foreseeable future. "The idea," he explains "would be that when you're 20 or 30, you would undergo treatment that would reprogram you—erase the aging [you've undergone to date]." That would "allow you not to age" in the usual sense. Barzilai admits that no therapy or technology capable of doing something like that yet exists. And it will not be easy to create it. "The rejuvenation of old to young is really difficult," he concedes. "But that doesn't mean we shouldn't want to try [to make it happen]."[3]

Cellular Senescence in the Aging Process

To find and implement the antiaging technologies that could make Sinclair's and Barzilai's antiaging scenarios a reality, science must establish what causes aging in the first place. Once a complete mystery, in the past half century geneticists and other researchers have begun to reveal some of the physical processes that drive the aging process. Among the mechanisms behind that process, they have found, is cellular senescence, essentially the limit to the number of times that a single cell can divide and remain viable and healthy. The maximum number of times that can happen, researchers have discovered, is somewhere between fifty and seventy. That threshold is called the Hayflick limit, named after Leonard Hayflick, author of *How and Why We Age* and a professor of anatomy at the University of California, San Francisco, School of Medicine. When a cell becomes senescent, it does not necessarily immediately die; but it does shut down and no longer functions the way it did in the past. Cellular senescence is crucial to aging because as one grows older the steady accumulation of senescent cells impedes the regeneration of healthy tissue to one degree or another.

Consider the stem cells in bone marrow. They produce immune cells, which are among the most vital cells in the body for good health and longevity. As we age, the bone marrow stem cells are slowly converted to a state of cellular senescence, which quite naturally leads to a diminished production of immune cells. With a weakened immune system, elderly adults are more prone to infections that younger adults can easily fight off. That is why infectious diseases such as pneumonia can be so deadly to older individuals.

Exactly why there is a limit to a cell's ability to divide and remain viable and healthy remains a medical mystery.

But a few reasons have been proposed. One of the most widely accepted hypotheses at present involves the telomeres within cells. Telomeres are extra sections of genetic material that exist at the ends of chromosomes. A simple analogy used by many scientists is that telomeres are like the plastic tips on shoelaces, which protect the rest of the lace. When someone cuts off one of those pieces of plastic, the shoelace it protected frays and can unravel. In a similar manner, the leading theory of the cause of senescence proposes that a cell's telomeres get shorter each time that cell divides. Eventually, the chromosomes run out of telomeres to protect them; hence, they can no longer function normally and therefore become senescent. Concurrently, over time a cell that repeatedly divides accumulates small amounts of DNA damage. Cells try to repair such damage and succeed in doing so to some extent. But when enough DNA damage occurs, the cell can become nonviable and senescent.

Longevity scientists want to find out how to prolong the productive life of a stem cell—or any healthy cell for that matter—both to help people better fend off diseases and to make them fight the aging process and live longer. One avenue involves boosting telomerase activity within cells. Telomerase is a protein that has sometimes been seen to naturally extend the length of some telomeres. According to experts, cells in which the length of the telomeres have increased demonstrated increased longevity. Current research is examining ways to activate telomerase with naturally occurring molecules delivered in drug treatments to slow down cell aging and hopefully prevent the occurrence of age-related diseases that might be accentuated by senescence.

Switching Genes On and Off

Another antiaging approach that researchers are currently examining involves dozens of known genes that appear to influence human longevity in one way or another. Some of these genes seem to increase longevity, while others seem to work against it. The goal is to find ways to control these genes so that the ones that promote longevity stay turned on while the ones that restrict longevity stay turned off. Switching genes on or off may—in addition to adhering to a healthier lifestyle—be one of several answers to prolonging the human life span in the near future.

In general, the longevity genes fall under three main categories: AMPK, mTOR, and sirtuins. Evidence suggests that AMPK genes promote longevity, and scientists have identified these genes as among the ones that oversee the metabolism of cells: that is, the way those cells change food into energy. A safe and inexpensive drug that activates AMPK—metformin—is currently available. Interestingly, it is prescribed by many doctors to treat diabetes, and research shows that people with diabetes who take metformin live longer than those who have diabetes and do not take that drug. Although more evidence and research are needed to verify this conclusion, the side effect of diabetes treatment provides circumstantial evidence of the potential antiaging effects of AMPK.

In contrast, the mTOR gene reduces longevity because when the gene is active, it is easier for a cell to enter a state of senescence. Aware of this effect, researchers have conducted studies in which they edited out mTOR from chromosomes to see what would happen to cells that no longer had it. They found that eliminating this gene prevented the onset of senescence, just as they had hoped would happen. Scientists have also found that even if the mTOR remains in place, losing weight and exercising regularly are natural ways to restrict the gene's activity and thereby slow down the aging process of some of the body's tissues.

Like AMPK, the third and last of the three gene types, sirtuins, promotes longevity. Much is still unknown about the functions of sirtuins, but they seem to play a role in regulating cells' energy production. It appears that sirtuins also ensure that genes that should not be turned on in certain cells are turned off. For this and other reasons, sirtuins seem to provide modest longevity benefits in various animals, including humans.

Turning Back the Cells' Biological Clocks

Targeted activation or deactivation of these longevity genes offers promise in significantly slowing down the aging process. However, many researchers feel that cellular-level antiaging efforts will not solely consist of manipulating genes in this manner. Instead, they say, it may well be within the reach of medical science to reverse the aging process. If successful, another approach would, in a sense, turn back the biological clocks of our cells. Longevity experts call this branch of antiaging research cellular reprogramming.

To reprogram cells, scientists have found that they must make those cells return to the state they were in when inside the developing embryo. This is accomplished on a regular basis in regenerative medicine when stem cells have their age reset backward almost to zero with the aid of the four Yamanaka factors. That sort of therapy usually takes place when someone's cells are manipulated in the lab and then transplanted back into the body. In contrast, cellular reprogramming is the effort to reverse aging by doing so in vivo; that is, directly inside the body of a living thing. This approach was first employed in a number of labs in the United States beginning in 2020. The Yamanaka factors were injected in liquid form directly into the blood, eyes, liver, and other parts of the bodies of mice and other animals so that large sections of tissue were affected at the same time in each case.

The results of these experiments were reported in several reputable journals, among them *Nature* and *Nature Aging*. Astonishingly, not only were the animals healed of various infirmities, they also appeared to revert to a younger, overall healthier state. Some of the mice, for example, were suffering from damaged retinal cells in their eyes before the experiment began. After receiving cellular reprogramming through injection, however, the rear sections of their eyes steadily healed and their sight was restored. At the same time, the mice exhibited a significantly more youthful appearance and higher energy levels. "We are elated," commented researcher Juan Carlos Belmonte of the Salk Institute for Biological Studies, "that we can use this approach . . . to slow down aging in normal animals. The technique is both safe and effective in mice [and other nonhumans]."[4]

Keep Stem Cells Young and Healthy

Two significant implications of cellular reprogramming derive from its ability to be deployed in vivo and from its effect on stem cells. First, cellular reprogramming within the body opens the door to a blanket antiaging therapy that could eventually target every cell in the human body. In other words, injecting Yamanaka factors into the blood of one or more organs ensures they will travel to every cell in the body. This is more efficient than the regenerative medicine practice of replacing old parts of the body just as we would replace old parts of a car. The second crucial implication of cellular re-programming is that it affects stem cells in addition to mature adult cells. Being able to keep stem cells young and healthy is important because they also age. Adult stem cells found in organs and tissues are still subject to DNA damage and epigenetic changes like mature cells are. Keeping adult stem cells healthy prevents them from becoming senescent stem cells. The more stem cells that are lost, the less regenerative potential the body has to heal inflammation and injury.

Despite these extremely positive developments in efforts to extend the human life span, one ongoing concern voiced by some experts is the potential for reduced or even poor quality of life for future people who live much longer than people do today. One such argument is that keeping people alive for hundreds of years might be more like a penalty than a gift, especially if along the way they suffer from physical pain or mental anguish. It is true that a long life span would be useless—or even merciless—if the individual is in constant pain from degenerative joint disease and back pain, cognitively impaired from Alzheimer's disease or other dementia, or suffering from a catalog of neurotic or psychotic disorders.

In response to that concern, other researchers point out that one of the major attractions of antiaging medicine is that it has the potential to target every cell in the human body. That includes cells in the joints, nerves, brain, and so forth. In this view, there is every reason to believe that the same techniques that will allow people to live far longer will also heal, or at least revitalize, their ailing body parts. Therefore, antiaging medicine such as cellular reprogramming has the potential to increase human life span while maintaining a favorable quality of life.

Living to Age 150, or Even 1,000?

The therapies of tomorrow discussed thus far hold the promise of extending human life expectancy and life span. In fact, it is likely that combinations of these therapies and others that are anticipated in the future may possibly enable humans to live even longer than 150 years. And taken to the extreme, perhaps in the far future (three or four centuries from now), science and medicine will have achieved such a state of dominion over disease and aging that a human being could be kept alive for several hundred years. Attaining an age beyond that is too difficult to predict at present because no one today can reasonably know whether some new technology that now appears purely fanciful might someday become commonplace.

That does not mean, of course, that all fantastic predictions about aging will be realized. In this regard, some people point to the SENS (Strategies for Engineered Negligible Senescence) Research Foundation, a facility for the study of longevity in Mountain View, California. Members of the staff there explore the use of regenerative medicine and other technologies that might allow humans to reverse or at least greatly slow down the aging process. What makes the SENS Research Foundation different from most facilities investigating human longevity is that several of its researchers are convinced that enormously long lifetimes—a thousand years or more—are not only possible but also within reach in the next few decades. In the words of the foundation's in-house science writer, Michael Rae:

> Once you take away ageing, it becomes open-ended. That doesn't mean you're immortal. You can still be murdered or hit by a catastrophic infection like Ebola, or die in a plane crash. But you are no longer going to be more vulnerable to disease and death. At that point, if you do the math on how unlikely it is to die, it gives a life expectancy of about 1,000 years. You can still die the next day, or live to 2,000 years. It becomes about what happens in your life.[5]

The majority of the world's longevity researchers feel that the SENS Research Foundation's aging predictions are unrealistic. They suggest that, although in theory it might be possible to develop the technologies to make such extreme longevity possible, it will likely be centuries before humanity reaches that high level of technical sophistication. More realistically, most experts think that 150 years will be the upper limit of the human lifetime. A far more important point, they say, is not how old one person might become, but rather how many people overall will be granted very long (and hopefully reasonably healthy) lives. The truth is that, thanks to myriad advances in medicine—especially knowledge of germs and the uses of vaccines and antibiotics, sanitation and clean drinking water, and discoveries made about aging—today far more people live past the ages of seventy, eighty, ninety, and one hundred than they did in all of human history. According to science writer Michael Eisenstein, "The United Nations estimates that there were 573,000 centenarians [people over the age of 100] alive worldwide in 2020—more than 20 times the number 50 years earlier. And hundreds of people reached the rarefied ranks of the supercentenarians, aged 110 or older, although demographers have validated the records of only a fraction of them."[6] Likewise, studies indicate that there are far more people who live past ninety, past eighty, and past seventy than ever before. These facts suggest that there is currently an ongoing upward trend of more and more people living longer.

Not only is this trend going to continue, as virtually every expert in the field agrees, it will noticeably speed up in the decades ahead. Indeed, "Science fiction has become science," says Greg Bailey, chief executive officer of the UK-based antiaging biotech company Juvenescence. Speaking of the speed of antiaging innovation, Bailey adds, "I think the world is going to be shocked." He likens the results of today's longevity research to early advances in human flight, saying,

> "In 1903, two brothers flew a glorified kite for 14 seconds, the Kitty Hawk. Fifteen years later they were flying planes in WWI, and 35 years later, the Germans had invented the jet. Sixty-five years later we landed a man on the moon. For robotics and for aging, divide that number by 10. That's how fast this is going to happen."[7]

Notes

1. Caroline Delbert, "Humans Could Live to Be 150, Science Says: But That's the Absolute Limit," *Popular Mechanics*, July 30, 2021. www.popularmechanics.com.

2. Quoted in Hannah Critchfield, "Is Aging a Disease? Treating It Like One Could Be Worth Trillions, Study Says," *Tampa Bay Times* (St. Petersburg, FL), July 15, 2021. www.tampabay.com.

3. Quoted in Eleanor Garth, "Nir Barzilai: 'Take Out the Noise and Focus on Tackling Aging,'" Longevity.Technology, May 5, 2022. https://longevity.technology.

4. Quoted in Genetic Engineering & Biotechnology News, "Aging Delayed in Mice Through Longer-Term Partial Reprogramming," March 8, 2022. www.genengnews.com.

5. Quoted in SENS Research Foundation, "British *Daily Mirror* Featured an Interview with SENS Research Foundation's Science Writer Michael Rae About the World's Richest Men Taking On the Longevity Challenge," November 21, 2021. www.sens.org.

6. Michael Eisenstein, "Does the Human Lifespan Have a Limit?," *Nature*, January 19, 2022. www.nature.com.

7. Quoted in Robin S. Jefferson, "'Extraordinary' Breakthroughs in Anti-Aging Research 'Will Happen Faster than People Think,'" *Forbes*, August 26, 2019. www.forbes.com.

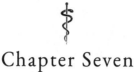

Chapter Seven

Reconstruction of

Consciousness

The antiaging therapies of tomorrow hold the promise of extending human life expectancy and life span. In fact, leading scientists anticipate that combinations of these therapies and others will eventually enable humans to live for a few hundred years. And taken to the extreme, perhaps in the far future, science and medicine will have advanced to the point that far longer lives might be possible.

However, even if scientific advancements turn this projection into a reality, there will remain one threat to human health and well-being that medical technology cannot resolve. This obstacle to achieving a sort of practical immortality stems from the randomness that exists in nature and everyday life. In fact, removing disease from the equation completely, we are left with the fact that merely being alive presents certain risk factors. Every day of our lives, there is a chance, however minuscule, of being hit by a car, falling down the stairs, being struck by lightning, or suffering from one of dozens of other unexpected negative events or circumstances.

For example, the CDC ranks accidents and unintentional injuries as the fourth leading cause of death in the United States. Add up all these incidentals, multiply them by the average human life expectancy, and one arrives at a contingency for personal adversity that cannot be ignored. Finally, consider the fact that in the future, humans will be living much longer lives and as a result will, simply by the law of averages, have a higher likelihood of experiencing some sort of reversal of fortune. The risk of random injury, accident, or death is therefore real, and if such tragedy strikes, the medical therapies might not remedy the situation.

Can Human Consciousness Be Preserved?

It should be emphasized, however, that these possible setbacks deriving from the randomness of life are, for the most part, physical in nature; that is, they most often involve damage of one kind or another to the body. As long as there is no injury to the brain, the mind will likely be unaffected; and some experts argue that the mind—or one's individual consciousness, with its memories and ability to perceive and reason—is what ultimately makes an individual unique. And some scientists argue that if one's consciousness can somehow be preserved for long periods of time—even if the body no longer functions as well as it once did—that person can in a very real sense defy the aging process. Journalist and science writer Simon Parkin asks:

> If you could save your mind like a comput-
> er's hard drive, would you? It's a question
> some hope to pose to us soon. They are the
> engineers working on the technology that
> will be able [to] create wholesale copies of
> our minds and memories that live on after
> we are burned or buried. If they succeed,
> it promises to have profound, and perhaps
> unsettling, consequences for the way we
> live, who we love and how we die.[1]

It is only natural to ask how the human mind might survive for long periods, including if the body were gone. In his remarks above, Parkin hints at an answer: namely, that the mind might somehow become part of a kind of computer interface. Indeed, several scientists have pro-posed that a human mind is made up of a highly com-plex collection of electrical impulses and that it might be transferable to some kind of digital format that can store it. This "mind uploading," a fairly new term many researchers have adopted for want of a more accurate descriptive term, is different from the previous therapies discussed in this book because it does not involve the application of chemical, genetic, or other medical ideas or practices or the treatment one would expect to receive in a hospital or clinic. Instead, artificially prolonging the existence of one's consciousness may eventually involve applying extremely sophisticated technologies, one of which involves computers and digital information. This concept is based on the fact that the brain appears to possess certain characteristics that are strikingly similar to those within the digital realm of a powerful computer. They both transmit information via electrical signaling and both can adapt, learn, and store memory. "Imagine that a person's brain could be scanned in great detail and recreated in a computer simulation," says Princeton University neuroscientist Michael Graziano.

> The person's mind and memories, emotions and personality would be duplicated. In effect, a new and equally valid version of that person would now exist, in a potentially immortal, digital form. This futuristic possibility is called mind uploading. The science of the brain and of consciousness increasingly suggests that mind uploading is possible. There are no laws of physics to prevent it. The technology is likely to be far in our future; it may be centuries before the

details are fully worked out, and yet given how much interest and effort is already directed towards that goal, mind uploading seems inevitable.[2]

The Complexities of the Human Mind

Comparisons of the human mind generated by the brain to a computer's circuitry are far from perfect. But as some experts point out, there are certain similarities. One is that a computer contains large numbers of individual pieces of information that are expressed as ones and zeros, and a human brain contains huge numbers of cells, called neurons, each with enormous numbers of connections to other cells. In both cases, electrical signals travel in circuitous ways, transmitting information at fantastic speeds. To get an idea of how amazingly complex this is within a human brain, consider the following excerpt from a 2022 article by Guillaume Thierry, a professor of neuroscience at Bangor University in Wales. Thierry describes a groundbreaking 2020 study by a team of researchers at the Allen Institute for Brain Science in Seattle, Washington, who mapped the 3-D structure of all the neurons existing within one cubic millimeter of a mouse's brain. "Within this minuscule cube of brain tissue, the size of a grain of sand," he states, the researchers counted more than 100,000 neurons and more than a billion connections between them. They managed to record the corresponding information on computers, including the shape and configuration of each neuron and connection, which required two petabytes, or two million gigabytes of storage. And to do this, their automated microscopes had to collect 100 million images of 25,000 slices of the minuscule sample continuously over several months. Now if this is what it takes to store the full physical information of neurons and their connections in one cubic millimeter of mouse brain, you can perhaps imagine that the collection of this information from the human brain is not going to be a walk in the park![3]

Indeed, Thierry's description of the complexities of the tiny building blocks of what constitutes a conscious human mind demonstrates how difficult it will be to digitalize and store the mind of a single human being. Yet when one considers how far computer and digital technology has advanced in the past thirty years alone, surely it is not beyond the realm of possibility that the advanced computer systems that will be available in 50

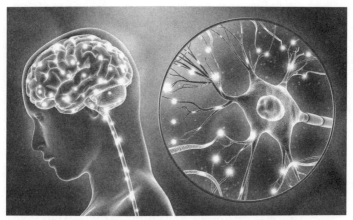

The human brain consists of huge numbers of cells called neurons. Neurons provide the pathways for the brain to send information back and forth to the body at fantastic speeds much like a computer's circuitry processes information.

or 100 or 150 years will have such masterful capability. And if indeed the information stored within a person's brain via its many neuronal connections can someday be scanned and stored inside a supercomputer, that mind will have defeated the aging process for some unknown length of time (perhaps as long as that given computer still functions and is maintained).

The Coming of Brain-Computer Interfaces

Granted, scientists are relatively far off from making mind uploading a reality. However, advances in brain-computer interfaces demonstrate the feasibility of linking a human brain to a computer. Although the following is not an example of reconstructing consciousness per se, it does suggest the overall trend toward melding mind with computer. Neuralink, a neural interface technology company founded by Elon Musk (b. 1971), the well-known entrepreneur, futurist, transhumanist, engineer, and inventor, focuses on building brain-computer devices that link human brains to computers. The goal of the company is to construct a brain implant that allows the user to control technology in the outside world by just thinking about it. Within the realm of science fiction, this may be known as mind control. Within the neurotechnology world, it is known as a brain-computer interface.

The clinical applications of such a technology would be game changing. Those with paralyzing spinal cord lesions could simply think of a text and the interface would send those neuronal signals to a phone where the text would write itself in real time. Such a sophisticated technological system would also be able to use thoughts to control prosthetics for those with amputations.

The truly exciting implication of such future brain-computer interfaces is that if this technology becomes a reality, it will represent the first bridge that has connected human brains with computers. Computers will be able to understand and interpret our thoughts. If connecting the brain to a computer is feasible, then the next step might be to meld the two together with mind-uploading technology.

Assuming mind uploading becomes a reality, what might that look like for those interested in continuing their consciousness digitally? Three plausible scenarios currently accepted by scientists and futurists have been proposed. They all begin with individuals living a normal life. Toward the end of their physical life or after an unexpected accident-causing death, their brain is scanned to extract their personality, memories, skills, and anything else that is stored there. The copied brain data is then uploaded into a computer.

The World Within a Digital Universe

From here, we can diverge into the first of the three potential scenarios, which involves living in a digital universe. This virtual world constructed inside a computer may be a simulation of real life or something entirely different. In a digital world, we would not be bound by the limitations of physics, so the possibilities of life would be endless. It is difficult to imagine ever getting bored in a world where anything is possible.

The second scenario involves taking our uploaded mind and transferring it into an avatar or cyborg, or in more conventional terms, a robot, albeit a very sophisticated one. We would still possess our mind, but we would be inhabiting an artificial body. In this scenario we would be able to continue to live in the real world within the body of this avatar. There would be a few different scenarios that might develop from this, of course, some of them not necessarily pleasant and others even a bit scary. As futurist and filmmaker Rob Merritt points out, for instance,

> If the company builds a robotic version of a human being does the company own them? It's their parts, their technology, their research, or does that person? Because supposedly they're human. What happens if it turns out you can take a brain pattern and make multiple versions of it, and you can make five versions of the same person? Which one's the real one? . . . If you destroy one of these things did you commit murder? Or did you just damage property? . . . I mean, all of a sudden you ask one question which leads to ten more, which leads to ten more, and you're like oh my god, this is huge![4]

The final scenario is perhaps the most interesting. As described by Michio Kaku, the popular theoretical physicist, in a video series by Big Think, believes our uploaded consciousness will not be limited to this world alone. "I think we're going to shoot [our digital mind] into outer space," he says. That is, if we can upload our minds, then we will be existing as code, just [ones and zeros] inside a computer. We will be data and information. There is technically no reason why we would not be able to send that data through space. In the future perhaps this will be to the moon or different planets where we can continue to live outside of the confines of Earth. Kaku takes it a step further in suggesting that alien life forms have already beaten us to this technology and that their "beams of consciousness"[5] are flying past us on Earth without us even knowing.

The Logical Next Step in Human Evolution?

It must be noted that a major impediment to mind-uploading technology is our minimal understanding of consciousness. Scientists and philosophers have debated and continue to debate what is meant by consciousness. An all-purpose definition is the state of being aware and responsive to one's surroundings. However, the seminal question still remains unanswered: How does a conscious thought find its way out of a pile of brain tissue? In the meantime, we can probe other questions such as whether reproducing consciousness will be transmitting our own selves into a digital world or creating an exact replica of ourselves instead. This technology would be useless in extending lives if it clones a mind instead of transferring it. Questions like this are difficult to answer until we have a deeper understanding of consciousness itself, and that will only come with time and more research.

Despite the technological obstacles that science will have to navigate to make mind uploading a reality, many argue that it is the logical next step in human evolution. Throughout history humans have constantly turned to medicine to solve their health problems and increase their life expectancy. Perhaps in the future, uploading one's mind to a computer server may be considered a common aspect of medicine. Since medicine as we know it can protect us from death only to a point, mind uploading may be the sole option for those who wish to truly live forever. Shedding our physical bodies and accepting a digital life may seem scary and intimidating, but in the future this may become a normal part of everyday life, especially if it promises immortality.

Notes

1. Simon Parkin, "Back-Up Brains: The Era of Digital Immortality," BBC, January 22, 2015. www.bbc.com.
2. Michael Graziano, "What Happens If Your Mind Lives Forever on the Internet?," *The Guardian* (Manchester, UK), October 20, 2019. www.theguardian.com.
3. Guillaume Thierry, "When Will I Be Able to Upload My Brain to a Computer?," The Conversation, June 9, 2022. https://theconversation.com.
4. Quoted in Aaron Horn, "Human Brains in Robot Bodies: An Interview with Filmmaker Rob Merritt," NewBoCo, October 9, 2017. https://newbo.co.

5. Quoted in Big Think, *Immortality: Can We Up-load Human Consciousness?* YouTube, 2021. www.youtube.com/watch?v=E3FRtUTFZuk&t=475s.

Epilogue

Humanity's current life expectancy is approximately twice that of our early ancestors whose flourishing cities dotted the fertile banks of the river valleys of the ancient Near East six millennia ago. And it would seem clear that medical science today is committed to an extended trajectory that will eventually bring the entire human race to the outermost boundaries of its potential life span. From anecdotal references on TV commercials, to articles in national journals, to published works by prominent medical scientists, living 150 years (and even more) is being bandied about today as very achievable, even before this current century passes into history.

Indeed, the medicine of tomorrow described in *Defying Death: Medicine's Journey Toward Immortality* contains the promise of adding decades and even centuries to our lives, quite possibly within the lifetime of some who are now reading these words. What was clearly perceived as unadulterated science fiction not very long ago is currently being developed in laboratories and research facilities around the globe. This serves as an indispensable reminder that Part II of this book remains unfinished. The science driving the medicine of tomorrow will continue to expand, producing innumerable changes and advances that are unimaginable today but will in time inevitably propel longevity to new lengths. And it just may happen that somewhere in the future there will be other unfinished books whose pages will direct their readers to a door on which are deeply etched these beckoning words: *Welcome. Forever Awaits You.*

Glossary

anaerobic: Capable of thriving without free oxygen; most often applied to certain types of bacteria.

antibiotic: A medicine that kills or inhibits the growth of bacteria.

antiseptic: A germ-killing agent.

bacteriology: The study of bacteria.

cardiology: The study of the heart and cardiovascular system and the diseases that can affect them.

chromosomes: Long chains of genes within a cell's nucleus.

CRISPR: A molecular tool used to edit DNA. The acronym stands for *clustered regularly interspaced short palindromic repeats*.

DNA: The genetic material that determines the various characteristics of living things. The letters stand for *deoxyribonucleic acid*.

empiricism: The concept that all knowledge derives from detection by the senses.

epigenetics: The study of how human behaviors and the environment cause changes in the expression of genes.

four bodily humors: Throughout the Middle Ages, the practice of medicine was predicated upon the theory of the four humors (blood, black bile, yellow bile, and phlegm). The state of good health was dependent upon the four humors remaining in balance with each other as they circulated throughout the body.

genes: Basic units of heredity found within the DNA of all cells.

genetics: The study of heredity.

germ theory: The concept, emerging in the nineteenth century, that disease is principally caused by microbes.

Hayflick limit: The maximum number of times that a single cell can divide.

iPSCs: Cells that start out highly specialized but are reprogrammed, allowing them to turn into any cell in the body. The letters stand for *induced pluripotent stem cells.*

life expectancy: The average amount of time a person or other living thing is expected to live.

metamorphosis: A complete change or transformation in form.

miasma: A nonexistent poisonous fog or vapor that doctors used to believe caused many diseases.

microbiology: The study of microbes, or germs.

mind uploading: The still-futuristic process by which a person's consciousness might one day be digitized and entered into a computer.

mutation: A random change in one or more genes that could lead to some of a person's or animal's physical traits being altered.

natural selection: The evolutionary process by which various animal and plant species slowly but steadily change and adapt to their environment.

nephrology: The study of the kidneys and the diseases that can affect them.

nucleotides: The molecular building blocks of DNA.

panacea: A supposed fix or cure-all for a disease or negative situation.

pluripotent cells: Undifferentiated cells that exist primarily within the embryo.

proteins: The individual building blocks of the body's tissues.

pulmonology: The study of the lungs and respiratory system.

regenerative medicine: A collection of technologies whose common goal is to replace damaged tissue with functional tissue.

senescence: The process of aging, or growing older. Or more specifically, the term can describe the state cells enter when they are no longer capable of dividing; in that state they are said to be senescent.

stem cells: Cells that can continue to divide a number of times to replenish the cells that die within bodily tissues.

stereolithography: The original and technical name for 3-D printing.

therapeutics: A general name for medical treatments.

transhumanist: Someone who advocates enhancing the human condition by using technologies that increase longevity.

Yamanaka factors: Microscopic substances that can induce ordinary cells to become iPSCs.

Works Consulted

Stuart Armstrong, *Smarter than Us: The Rise of Machine Intelligence*. Berkeley, CA: Machine Intelligence Research Institute, 2014.

Anthony Atala et al., eds., *Principles of Regenerative Medicine*. Cambridge, MA: Academic Press, 2018.

Elizabeth Blackburn and Elissa Epel, *The Telomere Effect: A Revolutionary Approach to Living Younger, Healthier, Longer*. London: Orion, 2017.

William Bynum, *The History of Medicine: A Very Short Introduction*. Oxford: Oxford University Press, 2008.

Nessa Carey, *The Epigenetics Revolution*. New York: Columbia University Press, 2013.

Logan Clendening, ed., *Sourcebook of Medical History*. New York: Dover, 1960.

Dorothy H. Crawford, *Deadly Companions: How Microbes Shaped Our History*. New York: Oxford University Press, 2009.

Dorothy H. Crawford, *Viruses: A Very Short Introduction*. Oxford: Oxford University Press, 2018.

Charles Greene Cumston, *An Introduction to the History of Medicine*. New York: Dorset, 1987.

Aubrey De Grey with Michael Rae, *Ending Aging: The Rejuvenation Breakthroughs That Could Reverse Human Aging in Our Lifetime*. New York: St. Martin's, 2007.

Jennifer A. Doudna and Samuel H. Sternberg, *A Crack in Creation: Gene Editing and the Unthinkable Power to Control Evolution*. New York: Mariner, 2018.

Cath Ennis, *Introducing Epigenetics: A Graphic Guide*. London: Icon, 2017.

Madeleine P. Grant, *Louis Pasteur, Fighting Hero of Science*. London: Hassell Street, 2021.

Michael Greger with Gene Stone, *How Not to Die*. London: Pan, 2018.

Leonard Hayflick, *How and Why We Age*. New York: Ballantine, 1994.

Michio Kaku, *The Future of Humanity: Our Destiny in the Universe*. New York: Anchor, 2019.

Dmitry Kaminskiy, *Biomarkers of Human Longevity*. London: Deep Knowledge Group, 2021.

Lee Know, *Mitochondria and the Future of Medicine: The Key to Understanding Disease, Chronic Illness, Aging, and Life Itself*. Hartford, VT: Chelsea Green, 2018.

Ray Kurzweil, *The Singularity Is Near: When Humans Transcend Biology*. New York: Penguin, 2005.

Ray Kurzweil and Terry Grossman, *Transcend: Nine Steps to Living Well Forever*. New York: Rodale, 2009.

Bruno Leone, *Disease in History*. San Diego, CA: ReferencePoint, 2016.

Bruno Leone, *Origin: The Story of Charles Darwin*. Greensboro, NC: Morgan Reynolds, 2009.

Elisa Lottor, *The Miracle of Regenerative Medicine: How to Naturally Reverse the Aging Process*. Rochester, VT: Healing Arts, 2018.

Lois N. Magner, *A History of Medicine*. New York: Marcel Dekker, 1992.

James E. McClellan III and Harold Dorn, *Science and Technology in World History: An Introduction*. Baltimore: Johns Hopkins University Press, 2015.

Jamie Metzl, *Hacking Darwin: Genetic Engineering and the Future of Humanity*. Naperville, IL: Sourcebooks, 2020.

James K. Min, *3D Printing Applications in Cardiovascular Medicine*. Cambridge, MA: Academic Press, 2018.

Josh Mitteldorf, *Cracking the Aging Code*. New York: Flatiron, 2017.

Michel Morange, *A History of Biology*. Old Saybrook, CT: Tantor, 2021.

Christine Mummery, *Stem Cells: Scientific Fact and Fiction*. Cambridge, MA: Academic Press, 2021.

Neil Riordan, *Stem Cell Therapy: A Rising Tide: How Stem Cells Are Disrupting Medicine and Transforming Lives*. Self-Published, 2017.

Anil Seth, *Being You: A New Science of Consciousness*. London: Faber and Faber, 2021.

John Simmons, *The Scientific 100: A Ranking of the Most Influential Scientists, Past and Present*. Secaucus, NJ: Carol, 1996.

David Sinclair and Matthew D. LaPlante, *Lifespan: Why We Age and Why We Don't Have To*. New York: Harper Thorsons, 2021.

Jonathan Weiner, *Long for This World: The Strange Science of Immortality*. New York: HarperCollins, 2010.

David Wood, *The Abolition of Aging: The Forthcoming Radical Extension of Healthy Human Longevity*. London: Delta Wisdom, 2016.

Index

Page numbers in bold indicate illustrations.